Update on Endocrine Disorders During Pregnancy

Editors

RACHEL PESSAH-POLLACK
MARIA PAPALEONTIOU

ENDOCRINOLOGY AND METABOLISM CLINICS OF NORTH AMERICA

www.endo.theclinics.com

Consulting Editor
ROBERT RAPAPORT

September 2024 • Volume 53 • Number 3

ELSEVIER

1600 John F. Kennedy Boulevard • Suite 1800 • Philadelphia, Pennsylvania, 19103-2899

http://www.theclinics.com

ENDOCRINOLOGY AND METABOLISM CLINICS OF NORTH AMERICA Volume 53, Number 3
September 2024 ISSN 0889-8529, ISBN 978-0-443-29632-1

Editor: Taylor Hayes
Developmental Editor: Saswoti Nath

Endocrinology and Metabolism Clinics of North America (ISSN 0889-8529) is published quarterly by Elsevier Inc., 360 Park Avenue South, New York, NY 10010-1710. Months of issue are March, June, September, and December. Periodicals postage paid at New York, NY and additional mailing offices. Subscription prices are USD 419.00 per year for US individuals, USD 100.00 per year for US students and residents, USD 486.00 per year for Canadian individuals, USD 532.00 per year for international individuals, USD 100.00 per year for Canadian students/residents, and USD 245.00 per year for international students/residents. For institutional access pricing please contact Customer Service via the contact information below. To receive student/resident rate, orders must be accompanied by name of affiliated institution, date of term, and the signature of program/residency coordinator on institution letterhead. Orders will be billed at individual rate until proof of status is received. Foreign air speed delivery is included in all *Clinics* subscription prices. All prices are subject to change without notice. Orders, claims, and journal inquiries: Please visit our Support Hub page https://service.elsevier.com for assistance.

Reprints. For copies of 100 or more, of articles in this publication, please contact the Commercial Rights Department, Elsevier Inc., 360 Park Avenue South, New York, NY 10010-1710; phone: +1-212-633-3874; fax: +1-212-633-3820; E-mail: reprints@elsevier.com.

Endocrinology and Metabolism Clinics of North America is covered in *MEDLINE/PubMed (Index Medicus), EMBASE/Excerpta Medica, Current Contents/Clinical Medicine, Current Contents/Life Sciences, Science Citation Index, ISI/BIOMED, BIOSIS,* and *Chemical Abstracts.*

Contributors

CONSULTING EDITOR

ROBERT RAPAPORT, MD
Professor of Pediatrics, Division of Pediatric Endocrinology and Diabetes, Kravis
Children's Hospital, Emma Elizabeth Sullivan Professor of Pediatric Endocrinology and
Diabetes, The Icahn School of Medicine at Mount Sinai Director, Emeritus, New York, New
York, USA

EDITORS

RACHEL PESSAH-POLLACK, MD, FACE
Clinical Associate Professor, Department of Medicine, NYU Grossman School of
Medicine, Holman Division of Endocrinology, Diabetes and Metabolism, Lake Success,
New York, USA

MARIA PAPALEONTIOU, MD
Assistant Professor, Division of Metabolism, Endocrinology and Diabetes, Research
Assistant Professor, Institute of Gerontology, University of Michigan, Ann Arbor, Michigan,
USA

AUTHORS

RICHARD J. AUCHUS, MD, PhD
Professor, Departments of Pharmacology and Internal Medicine, Division of Metabolism,
Endocrinology and Diabetes, University of Michigan, Ann Arbor, Michigan, USA

JOHN P. BILEZIKIAN, MD
Professor of Medicine and Pharmacology, College of Physicians & Surgeons, Division of
Endocrinology, Department of Medicine, Vagelos College of Physicians and Surgeons,
Columbia University, New York, New York, USA

ADI COHEN, MD, MHS
Associate Professor, Division of Endocrinology, Professor of Medicine at CUMC,
Department of Medicine, Columbia University, College of Physicians & Surgeons, New
York, New York, USA

CHRYSOULA DOSIOU, MD, MS
Clinical Professor, Medical Director of the Thyroid Eye Clinic, Division of Endocrinology,
Department of Internal Medicine, Stanford University School of Medicine, Stanford,
California, USA

AOIFE M. EGAN, MB, BCH, PhD
Associate Professor, Division of Endocrinology, Diabetes and Metabolism, Department of
Medicine, Mayo Clinic, Rochester, Minnesota, USA

MARY ELIZABETH FINO, MD
Assistant Professor, Director, Oocyte Donation and 3rd Party Reproduction, Associate Director, Fellowship in Reproductive Endocrinology and Infertility, Division of Reproductive Endocrinology and Infertility, Department of Obstetrics and Gynecology, New York University Langone Prelude Fertility Center, New York, New York, USA

MARIA FLESERIU, MD
Professor and Director, OHSU Pituitary Center; Professor, Department of Medicine, Division of Endocrinology, Diabetes and Clinical Nutrition, Oregon Health & Science University, Department of Neurological Surgery, Pituitary Center, Oregon Health & Science University, Portland, Oregon, USA

MONICA LIVIA GHEORGHIU, MD, PhD
Professor, Department of Clinical Endocrinology IV, Carol Davila University of Medicine and Pharmacy Bucharest, CI Parhon National Institute of Endocrinology, Bucharest, Romania

MICHELE B. GLODOWSKI, MD
Clinical Instructor, Division of Endocrinology, Diabetes and Metabolism, Department of Medicine, New York University Langone Health, New York, New York, USA

IRA J. GOLDBERG, MD
Junior Professor of Endocrinology, Department of Medicine, New York University Grossman School of Medicine, Director, Holman Division of Endocrinology, Diabetes and Metabolism, New York University Grossman School of Medicine, New York, New York, USA

KEERTHANA HARIDAS, MBBS
Fellow, Division of Endocrinology, Diabetes and Metabolism, Department of Medicine, University of California Los Angeles David Geffen School of Medicine, Division of Endocrinology, Diabetes and Metabolism, Department of Medicine, Veterans Affairs Greater Los Angeles Healthcare System, Los Angeles, California, USA

ADRIANA G. IOACHIMESCU, MD, PhD
Professor, Department of Medicine, Division of Endocrinology and Molecular Medicine, Medical College of Wisconsin, Department of Neurosurgery, Medical College of Wisconsin, HUB for Collaborative Medicine, Milwaukee, Wisconsin, USA

IRENE Y. JUNG, BA
Research Technician, New York University Grossman School of Medicine, New York, New York, USA

ANGELA M. LEUNG, MD, MSc
Associate Professor, Division of Endocrinology, Diabetes and Metabolism, Associate Professor, Department of Medicine, University of California Los Angeles David Geffen School of Medicine, Division of Endocrinology, Diabetes and Metabolism, Department of Medicine, Veterans Affairs Greater Los Angeles Healthcare System, Los Angeles, California, USA

CAROL J. LEVY, MD, CDCES
Professor, Department of Medicine and Obstetrics, Division of Endocrinology, Diabetes, and Metabolism, The Icahn School of Medicine at Mount Sinai, New York, New York, USA

SPYRIDOULA MARAKA, MD, MS
Associate Professor of Medicine, Division of Endocrinology, Diabetes and Metabolism, Department of Internal Medicine, University of Askansas for Medical Sciences, Chief, Section of Endocrinology, Medicine Service, Central Arkansas Veterans Healthcare System, Little Rock, Arkansas, USA

ALON Y. MAZORI, MD
Fellow, Division of Endocrinology, Diabetes, and Metabolism, The Icahn School of Medicine at Mount Sinai, New York, New York, USA

SNEHA MOHAN, MBBS
Fellow, Division of Endocrinology, Diabetes and Metabolism, Department of Medicine, Mayo Clinic, Rochester, Minnesota, USA

YASAMAN MOTLAGHZADEH, MPH, MD
Clinical Assistant Professor, Division of Endocrinology, Gerontology and Metabolism, Department of Medicine, Stanford University School of Medicine, Palo Alto, California, USA

CARLOS M. PARRA, MD
Reproductive Endocrinology and Infertility Fellow, Division of Reproductive Endocrinology and Infertility, Department of Obstetrics and Gynecology, New York University Langone Prelude Fertility Center, New York, New York, USA

NICOLE REISCH, MD
Professor, Department of Medicine IV, Institute for Endocrinology, Diabetology and Metabolism, Ludwig Maximilian University of Munich, Germany

EMILY A. ROSENBERG, MD
Assistant Professor, Division of Endocrinology, Diabetes, and Metabolic Diseases, Medical University of South Carolina, Charleston, South Carolina, USA

TAMLYN SASAKI, BS
University of Hawaii John A. Burns School of Medicine, Honolulu, Hawaii, USA

DARIA SCHATOFF, MD
Endocrinology Fellow, New York University Grossman School of Medicine, New York, New York, USA

ELLEN W. SEELY, MD
Director of Clinical Research, Professor, Department of Medicine, Division of Endocrinology, Diabetes, and Hypertension, Brigham and Women's Hospital, Harvard Medical School, Boston, Massachusetts, USA

DEBORAH E. SELLMEYER, MD
Clinical Professor, Division of Endocrinology, Gerontology and Metabolism, Department of Medicine, Stanford University School of Medicine, Palo Alto, California, USA

MADELINE K. XIN, BA, MD, PhD
Trainee, NYU Grossman School of Medicine, New York, New York, USA

CATHERINE D. ZHANG, MD
Assistant Professor, Department of Medicine, Division of Endocrinology and Molecular Medicine, Medical College of Wisconsin, HUB for Collaborative Medicine, Milwaukee, Wisconsin, USA

Contents

> The care of pregnant individuals with type 1 diabetes mellitus has experienced significant advancements in recent years. Preconception counseling has re-emerged as a core dimension of management. Continuous glucose monitoring plays an increasingly useful and beneficial role in gestational glycemic monitoring, a practice informed by improved maternofetal outcomes. While studies have not shown that continuous subcutaneous insulin infusion is superior to multiple daily injections of insulin for glycemic control, recent work has signaled that hybrid closed-loop systems with pregnancy-specific targets could meaningfully improve glycemic control and potentially ameliorate maternofetal outcomes while reducing self-care burden.

> Hyperglycemia in pregnancy due to pre-existing Type 2 diabetes mellitus (T2DM) and gestational diabetes mellitus (GDM) is rising globally with increasing rates of risk factors for metabolic disease. This review summarizes current evidence and recommendations from national and international guidelines for diagnosis and management of T2DM and GDM to optimize maternal and neonatal outcomes.

> This review summarizes the diagnosis and management of thyrotoxicosis in pregnancy. The diagnostic clinical and biochemical considerations used to distinguish the various etiologies of hyperthyroidism from appropriate physiologic changes during pregnancy will be outlined. Finally, the review will discuss the risks and benefits of available options for the treatment of thyrotoxicosis during pregnancy, to mitigate the risks of fetal hyperthyroidism.

Pregnancy is rare in women with Cushing's syndrome (CS), due to hyper-cortisolism-induced gonadotropin suppression and anovulation. Diagnosis of CS is hampered by physiological cortisol level increases during normal pregnancy; importantly abnormal cortisol secretion circadian rhythm could be diagnostic. Active CS is associated with considerable maternal and fetal complications. Second trimester surgery (pituitary or adrenal) is the main treatment option, however observation in mild cases has been suggested. Medical treatment, although not approved for use in pregnancy, may be considered, after careful discussion and balancing any benefits with potential risks and side-effects.

Hypercalcemia during pregnancy is a risk for adverse maternal and fetal consequences. Although primary hyperparathyroidism is by far the most common etiology of hypercalcemia in pregnancy, an array of other etiologies of hypercalcemia associated with pregnancy and lactation have been described. Parathyroidectomy continues to be the preferred treatment for primary hyperparathyroidism. Medical management options are limited.

This article reviews bone metabolism, bone mass, and bone structure changes expected during and after pregnancy and lactation, as well as the condition of pregnancy and lactation-associated osteoporosis (PLO)—a presentation with fragility fracture(s) in the context of these physiologic changes. Clinical implications of physiologic bone changes will be addressed, as will specific management considerations that apply to premenopausal women with PLO.

Many transgender and gender diverse (TGD) individuals will be considering gender-affirming treatments during their reproductive lifespan. These medically necessary treatments have a negative impact on reproductive potential. All TGD individuals should be counseled regarding fertility. Options for fertility preservation for individuals who have undergone puberty include mature oocyte, embryo, and sperm cryopreservation. In prepubertal individuals, ovarian tissue cryopreservation may be considered, but testicular tissue cryopreservation remains experimental only. While there have been advances in the technology and standardization of reproductive health care for this population, many gaps remain in our knowledge which require further research.

Practicing endocrinologists are likely to confront 2 major issues that occur with dyslipidemias during pregnancy. The most dramatic is the development of severe hypertriglyceridemia leading to acute pancreatitis. The second is the approach to treatment of familial hypercholesterolemia, a common genetic disorder. This article reviews the normal physiology and the pathophysiology of lipoproteins that occurs with pregnancy and then discusses the approaches to prevention and/or treatment of dyslipidemia in pregnancy with a focus on lifestyle and acceptable drug therapies.

ENDOCRINOLOGY AND METABOLISM CLINICS OF NORTH AMERICA

SERIES OF RELATED INTEREST

Medical Clinics
https://www.medical.theclinics.com
Primary Care: Clinics in Office Practice
https://www.primarycare.theclinics.com/

Foreword

Update on Endocrine Disorders During Pregnancy

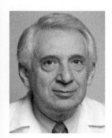

Robert Rapaport, MD
Consulting Editor

As of June 2024, PubMed yielded 6317 results on endocrine disorders during pregnancy. The first five publications listed were from the *Endocrinology and Metabolism Clinics of North America*, Volume 40, Issue 4, published in 2011 and guest edited by Drs Rachel Pessah-Pollack and Lois Jovanovic. The untimely death of Dr Jovanovic resulted in a multitude of tributes acknowledging her seminal contributions to the field of diabetes and pregnancy, notably the article "Gestational Diabetes Mellitus: New Evidence for the Continuing Challenge" from Volume 42 of Diabetes Care. Her impact on the field of health during pregnancy cannot be overestimated. We are therefore extremely pleased that Dr Rachel Pessah-Pollack has collaborated with Dr Maria Papaleontiou to produce an updated issue devoted to endocrine disorders during pregnancy. Their collaboration resulted in a timely, expert volume. It is fitting that the first article is devoted to the management of Type 1 Diabetes, given the incredible advances in diabetes management worldwide. Thyroid disorders, including hyperthyroidism, subclinical hypothyroidism, autoimmunity, congenital adrenal hyperplasia, Cushing syndrome, calcium and lipid disorders, and prolactin excess, are addressed by leading authorities. Attention is also paid to bone health and blood pressure disorders that occur during pregnancy. Drs Pessah-Pollack and Papaleontiou have done an excellent job enlisting eminent faculty to document the latest medical advances that provide a state-of-the-art compendium on endocrine disorders during pregnancy.

Endocrinol Metab Clin N Am 53 (2024) xiii–xiv
https://doi.org/10.1016/j.ecl.2024.06.002
0889-8529/24/© 2024 Published by Elsevier Inc.

endo.theclinics.com

DISCLOSURE

The author has no conflicts of interest to disclose.

Robert Rapaport, MD
Icahn School of Medicine at Mount Sinai Director, Emeritus
Division of Pediatric Endocrinology and Diabetes
Kravis Children's Hospital at Mount Sinai
1468 Madison Ave 4th Floor
New York, NY 10029, USA

E-mail address:
robert.rapaport@mountsinai.org

Preface

Endocrine Disorders During Pregnancy

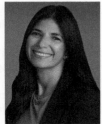
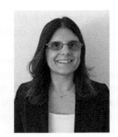

Rachel Pessah-Pollack, MD, FACE   Maria Papaleontiou, MD

Editors

It has been over ten years since the last publication of the *Endocrinology and Metabolism Clinics of North America* issue devoted to "Endocrine Disorders During Pregnancy." During this time, we have unfortunately lost an incredible physician, revered mentor, and pioneer in the field of diabetes in pregnancy, Dr Lois Jovanovic. Our knowledge and management of endocrine disorders during pregnancy have greatly improved with her research and immense dedication to advancing care for all women with diabetes during pregnancy. We devote this issue to the memory of Dr Lois Jovanovic and hope others will continue in her path of seeking new information and the best treatments for both mothers and children. We view pregnancy as a continuum, starting with preconception planning, continuing with gestation of the fetus, and culminating in the postpartum period.

For this issue, we have carefully selected topics of interest to a wide range of subspecialties primarily within adult endocrinology, but also managed by other specialists, including cardiologists, obstetricians, and reproductive endocrinologists. Distinguished experts from diverse settings provide a contemporary overview of these topics as they directly relate to patient care, incorporating the challenge of diagnosing endocrine disorders during pregnancy, which is often camouflaged by the normal symptoms and disorders seen during pregnancy.

Endocrinol Metab Clin N Am 53 (2024) xv–xvii
https://doi.org/10.1016/j.ecl.2024.06.001
0889-8529/24/© 2024 Published by Elsevier Inc.

Patients with type 1 diabetes face unique issues preconception and during pregnancy, and the article by Drs Mazori and Levy provides insight into these considerations. With the surge in cases of newly diagnosed type 2 diabetes mellitus in recent years, Drs Egan and Mohan specifically address pregestational diabetes and highlight the challenges of treatment both before and during pregnancy.

Thyroid disorders during pregnancy remain a "hot" topic of interest to clinicians. Dr Haridas, Ms Sasaki, and Dr Leung provide a comprehensive review regarding evaluation and management of thyrotoxicosis during pregnancy, highlighting the importance of multidisciplinary management. Drs Maraka and Dosiou address thyroid autoimmunity in pregnancy and delve into the debate of whether to treat subclinical hypothyroidism during pregnancy.

Dr Seely and Dr Rosenberg expertly discuss new approaches to diagnosing and treating hypertension in pregnancy, a topic of interest not only to endocrinologists but also to primary care physicians, cardiologists, and obstetricians.

The pituitary and adrenal glands play an integral role in the preconception, pregnancy, and postpartum periods, and their management depends on appropriately understanding the physiologic changes that occur during these periods. Addressing recent advances and increasing evidence in the field, Drs Reisch and Auchus tackle the management of congenital adrenal hyperplasia during pregnancy; Drs Ioachimescu and Zhang discuss the pathophysiology and evaluation of prolactinomas both before and during pregnancy, and how the treatment differs compared with the nonpregnant state, and Drs Gheorghiu and Fleseriu raise awareness regarding detection, diagnosis, and timely management of Cushing syndrome in pregnancy.

In addition, Drs Sellmeyer, Motlaghzadeh, and Bilezikian provide significant insight on the challenges of evaluation and management of hypercalcemia during pregnancy (often with symptoms mimicking normal symptoms of pregnancy), while Dr Cohen aptly addresses the topic of pregnancy-related bone loss and when treatment is needed versus monitoring.

Bringing attention to the reproductive health considerations in the transgender population ensures that the specific needs of this population are adequately addressed in order to improve patient care and experience. Dr Glodowski, Dr Parra, Ms Xin, and Dr Fino masterfully highlight many of the issues that should be considered regarding fertility preservation in transgender and gender diverse people. Finally, Dr Schatoff, Ms Jung, and Dr Goldberg skillfully discuss the challenges in hyperlipidemia management during pregnancy, highlighting recent advances in the field.

Owing to our colleagues' dedication, expertise, interest, and enthusiasm for this issue, it has been a privilege to serve as guest editors. We trust you will find these articles timely, informative, and enlightening, and we hope that this issue will provide valuable insight to help in the care of pregnant women and delivery of healthy babies. We are extremely thankful to the editorial staff for their assistance and support in the preparation of this issue.

DISCLOSURES

Dr Pessah-Pollack: Advisor for Boehringer Ingelheim/Eli Lilly. Maria Papaleontiou have no conflicts of interest to disclose.

Rachel Pessah-Pollack, MD, FACE
Department of Medicine
NYU Grossman School of Medicine
Holman Division of Endocrinology
Diabetes & Metabolism
1999 Marcus Avenue
Lake Success, NY 11042, USA

Maria Papaleontiou, MD
Division of Metabolism, Endocrinology and Diabetes
University of Michigan
North Campus Research Complex
2800 Plymouth Road
Building 16, Room 453S
Ann Arbor, MI 48109, USA

E-mail addresses:
Rpessahpollack@gmail.com (R. Pessah-Pollack)
mpapaleo@med.umich.edu (M. Papaleontiou)

Updates in the Management of Type 1 Diabetes in Pregnancy

Alon Y. Mazori, MD[a,1], Carol J. Levy, MD, CDCES[b,*]

KEYWORDS

- Type 1 diabetes • Pregnancy • Maternal/fetal outcomes
- Continuous glucose monitoring • Insulin • Insulin pump

KEY POINTS

- Pregnancies complicated by type 1 diabetes mellitus display an increased risk of maternal complications (eg, severe hypoglycemia, pre-eclampsia, cesarean delivery) and neonatal adverse events (eg, perinatal mortality, congenital malformations, hypoglycemia requiring neonatal intensive care unit admission).
- Gestational changes in insulin resistance confer an increased risk of hypoglycemia in the first trimester and hyperglycemia in subsequent trimesters.
- Preconception care should ensure that individuals of reproductive potential understand glycemic and health goals prior to pregnancy and review schedules for the monitoring of retinopathy, kidney disease, and hypertension.
- Continuous glucose monitoring (CGM) use in pregnancy, particularly real-time CGM, improves glycemic control and maternal and neonatal outcomes while lowering self-care burden in a cost-saving manner.
- Further research on pregnancy-specific hybrid closed-loop systems is necessary; off-label use can be considered in select individuals and experienced providers after careful discussion of risks, benefits, and alternatives, as well as strategies to optimize pump use and algorithms.

INTRODUCTION

Type 1 diabetes mellitus (T1D) is a disorder characterized by absolute insulin deficiency resulting from autoimmune destruction of pancreatic β-cells. While research

[a] Division of Endocrinology, Diabetes, and Metabolism, The Icahn School of Medicine at Mount Sinai, 1 Gustave L. Levy Place, New York, NY 10029, USA; [b] Division of Endocrinology, Diabetes, and Metabolism, The Icahn School of Medicine at Mount Sinai, 1 Gustave L. Levy Place, Box 1055, New York, NY 10029, USA
[1] Present address: 78 Crabtree Lane, Tenafly, NJ, 07670.
* Corresponding author.
E-mail address: carol.levy@mssm.edu

Endocrinol Metab Clin N Am 53 (2024) 321–333
https://doi.org/10.1016/j.ecl.2024.05.001
endo.theclinics.com

into treatments to cure or delay the progression of T1D is ongoing, insulin remains the core therapy.

Tighter pregnancy-specific maternal glycemic targets combine with gestational changes in insulin sensitivity and action profiles to raise the complexity of management of T1D for both the mother and fetus. As pregnancy progresses, lipolysis is accelerated, hepatic gluconeogenesis augmented, and insulin resistance in peripheral tissues increased. Consequently, insulin sensitivity dynamically changes during each trimester.[1,2] Insulin resistance falls over the course of the first trimester, thereby increasing the risk of maternal hypoglycemia.[1–3] The second and third trimesters, in contrast, exhibit progressively rising insulin resistance with resultant postprandial hyperglycemia.[1,2] Other complicating factors include increasingly delayed insulin absorption and gastric emptying with advancing gestation.[4]

Gestational insulin resistance potentiates maternal hyperglycemia, which confers an elevated risk of severe hypoglycemia, pre-eclampsia (PE), and cesarean delivery in pregnancies complicated by T1D.[2,3,5] In one nationwide, prospective cohort study[6] of 323 women with T1D in the Netherlands, the risk of PE was 12 fold greater than the general population (12.7% in T1D vs 1.05% nationally), and the risk of cesarean delivery was 3.7 fold greater (44.3% in T1D vs 12.0% nationally). Similar results were observed in larger nationwide studies in Denmark[7] and Taiwan.[8] The risk of neonatal complications is also higher, particularly congenital malformations, perinatal mortality, large for gestational age (LGA), and neonatal hypoglycemia requiring neonatal intensive care unit (NICU) admission.[5] A nationwide, prospective study in Denmark[7] estimated the risk of congenital malformations to be nearly double that of the general population (5.0% in T1D vs 2.8% nationally), and 3 nationwide cohort studies[6–8] calculated the risk of perinatal mortality to be 4 fold higher. Moreover, enhanced lipolysis in pregnancy engenders a ketogenic state that predisposes to diabetic ketoacidosis (DKA), which increases the risk of fetal loss to 10%, emergency cesarean delivery to 40%, and NICU admission to 52%.[6,9]

The chief obstacle to maternal glycemic control is achieving optimal pregnancy-specific glycemic control prior to and throughout pregnancy while balancing the risks of hypoglycemia and hyperglycemia and self-care burden. Beyond the difficulties posed by gestational metabolic changes, fewer than 40% of women with T1D receive preconception counseling (PCC) to help optimize maternal and fetal outcomes.[5,10] Self-monitoring of blood glucose (SMBG) through finger-stick testing and most recently real-time continuous glucose monitoring (rtCGM) have provided new opportunities to maximize glycemic control. Despite these tools, providers and patients still struggle whether to use multiple daily injections of insulin (MDI), continuous subcutaneous insulin infusion (CSII), or at times off-label use of hybrid closed-loop (HCL) systems to maximize maternal glycemic control.

PRECONCEPTION CARE

PCC provides an opportunity to optimize maternal and neonatal outcomes. A meta-analysis and systematic review found that PCC reduced the risk of congenital malformations by 71%, perinatal mortality by 54%, NICU admission by 25%, and preterm delivery by 15%.[11]

Two essential elements of PCC are to ensure all individuals of childbearing potential are aware of the ideal glycemic and health goals prior to pregnancy and to provide individualized discussion of available contraceptive methods. Explaining the materno-fetal consequences of gestational dysglycemia is crucial to minimize the risk of maternofetal complications (**Table 1**). Consensus guidelines[10] based on historical data

Table 1
Maternal and fetal/neonatal complications of dysglycemia in pregnancies complicated by type 1 diabetes

Maternal Complications	Fetal/Neonatal Complications
• Preterm delivery	• Neonatal hypoglycemia
• Pre-eclampsia	• Respiratory distress syndrome
• Severe hypoglycemia	• Admission to intensive care unit
• Miscarriage	• Fetal demise
• Cesarean delivery	• Macrosomia
• Accelerated or de novo retinopathy	• Shoulder dystocia
• Progression of nephropathy	• Large for gestational age
• Diabetic ketoacidosis	• Congenital malformations
	• Small for gestational age

Adapted from ElSayed NA, Aleppo G, Aroda VR, et al. 15. Management of Diabetes in Pregnancy: Standards of Care in Diabetes-2023. *Diabetes Care.* 2023;46(Suppl 1):S254-66; and Benhalima K, Beunen K, Siegelaar SE, et al. Management of type 1 diabetes in pregnancy: update on lifestyle, pharmacological treatment, and novel technologies for achieving glycaemic targets [published correction appears in *Lancet Diabetes Endocrinol.* 2023 Oct;11(10):e12]. Lancet Diabetes Endocrinol. 2023;11(7):490-508.

recommend a pregestational hemoglobin A1c (HbA1c) of 6.5% (47 mmol/L) to optimize maternal and neonatal outcomes; a stricter goal of 6.0% (42 mmol/L) can be pursued if hypoglycemia is avoided. Both pregnancy-specific SMBG and CGM glycemic targets should be introduced, as well as how the frequency of glucose monitoring can impact glycemic control, maternofetal outcomes, and options for insulin delivery. Ideally, pregnancy-specific glycemic targets should be attained 3 to 6 months prior to conception.

PCC also includes screening for and treatment of diabetes-related complications. Maternal hyperglycemia is associated with an elevated rate of progression of diabetic retinopathy,[5] which is the leading cause of irreversible blindness in individuals of reproductive age.[12] Accordingly, retinopathy screening should occur prior to pregnancy and during each trimester and be managed by a retinal specialist. Maternal hypertension and diabetes-related kidney disease warrant similar screening, as PE and preterm delivery can occur in up to 60% of pregnancies complicated by T1D with pre-existing hypertension or nephropathy.[13]

Additional recommendations for preconception care, including folate supplementation and screening for thyroid disorders, are included in **Box 1**.

FREQUENCY OF MONITORING DURING PREGNANCY

The frequency of endocrinology visits in pregnancy should consist of monthly visits (either in person or via telemedicine) combined with weekly communications regarding glucose levels to optimize insulin-dose titrations. Given the higher risk of maternal and neonatal complications, close obstetric follow-up should be provided by an obstetrician with expertise in pregnancies complicated by diabetes.

GLUCOSE MONITORING IN PREGNANCY
Continuous Glucose Monitoring

CGM, particularly rtCGM, is a useful technology for the management of diabetes in pregnancy. CGM not only enables providers to better assess glycemic patterns and tailor insulin therapy but also empowers patients to better understand the relationship

Box 1
Preconception care

General Topics
- Lifestyle optimization
  - Regular moderate exercise
  - Counseling for smoking cessation and alcohol abstinence
- Folate supplementation
- Increased frequency of follow-up with endocrinologist and obstetrician

Diabetes-specific Counseling
- Discussion of pregnancy-specific glycemic management
  - Gestational glycemic targets
  - Strategies for glucose monitoring (eg, continuous glucose monitoring)
  - Progressively delayed insulin absorption with advanced gestation
  - Method of insulin delivery (eg, injections vs insulin pump)
  - Diabetes-related complications
- Maternofetal impacts of gestational dysglycemia
- Overview of gestational metabolic changes
  - Risk of severe hypoglycemia in first trimester due to higher insulin sensitivity
  - Progressive insulin resistance in later pregnancy with risk of hyperglycemia
  - Ketogenic nature of pregnancy with elevated risk of diabetic ketoacidosis
- Review of carbohydrate counting
- Preferential intake of carbohydrates with low glycemic indices

Medication Review
- Diabetes: all off-label antihyperglycemic agents
- Blood pressure:
  - Angiotensin-converting enzyme inhibitors
  - Angiotensin II receptor blockers
  - Diuretics
- Dyslipidemia: statins

Screening Tests
- Thyroid function tests
- Lipid panel
- Prior to and throughout pregnancy:
  - Retinopathy: dilated eye examination
  - Nephropathy: urine protein-to-creatinine ratio
  - Neuropathy: monofilament examination

Genetic Screening
- Cystic fibrosis
- Sickle cell anemia
- Tay–Sachs disease
- Thalassemia

Screening for Infectious Diseases
- Human immunodeficiency virus
- Neisseria gonorrhea
- Chlamydia trachomatis
- Hepatitis C

Immunizations
- Rubella
- Varicella
- Hepatitis B
- Influenza

Adapted from ElSayed NA, Aleppo G, Aroda VR, et al. 15. Management of Diabetes in Pregnancy: Standards of Care in Diabetes-2023. *Diabetes Care.* 2023;46(Suppl 1):S254-66.

between glycemic targets and patterns in nutrition, exercise, and insulin dosing. CGMs temporally dynamic nature prompted the development of consensus guidelines for pregnancy-specific, CGM-based glycemic goals.[14] **Box 2** outlines these definitions and recommendations for pregnancy-specific time in range (psTIR), pregnancy-specific time above range (psTAR), and pregnancy-specific time below range (psTBR).

The landmark CONCEPTT[15] trial was an open-label, multicenter, and international randomized controlled trial that enrolled 314 participants in the first trimester. Participants were randomized to either SMBG alone or SMBG and rtCGM (Medtronic Guardian REAL-Time or MiniMed Minilink system). For the primary outcome of HbA1c decrement between randomization and 34 weeks of gestation, rtCGM use was associated with a greater difference (-0.54% vs -0.35%; $P = .0372$), which persisted after adjusting for potential confounders. rtCGM use was also associated with a greater HbA1c decrement between randomization and 24 weeks of gestation (-0.67% vs -0.52%; $P = .0374$), greater psTIR (68% vs 61%; $P = .0034$), and lower psTAR (27% vs 32%; $P = .0279$). psTBR, however, was similar between the 2 groups (3% vs 4%; $P = .10$). More importantly, rtCGM use was linked to less LGA (53% vs 69%; $P = .0210$), neonatal hypoglycemia requiring intravenous dextrose (15% vs 28%; $P = .0250$), NICU admission (27% vs 43%; $P = .0157$), and duration of NICU admission (3.1 vs 4.0 days; $P = .0091$). Such reductions of neonatal complications were accompanied by unchanged frequencies of DKA, severe hypoglycemia, PE, preterm delivery, and cesarean delivery.

The advantages of CGM use highlighted in CONCEPTT aligned with the findings of the smaller observational study LOIS-P.[2] Based in the United States, this multicenter study of 25 individuals examined participants who used CSII and were trained to combine SMBG with a Dexcom G6 rtCGM. Participants with at least one maternal complication (eg, gestational hypertension, PE, polyhydramnios, or preterm labor) had lower psTIR (49% vs 66%; $P = .001$). Lower psTIR was also noted among women whose children required NICU admission (52% vs 64%; $P = .05$). LGA, however, was not linked to psTIR.

Secondary analyses of CONCEPTT provided useful insights into additional benefits of rtCGM use. One study[16] leveraged functional data analysis to isolate temporal differences in 24 hour glucose profiles. The authors found that the CONCEPTT participants randomized to rtCGM exhibited higher daytime psTIR than those allocated to SMBG alone (67.6% vs 61.3%) and lower daytime psTAR (27.9% vs 33.1%). These findings prompted the hypothesis that the improved neonatal outcomes noted in the CGM group were connected to the reduced fetal exposure to daytime maternal hyperglycemia. In addition, the temporal analysis identified that women in the CGM

Box 2
Continuous glucose monitoring-based pregnancy-specific glycemic targets

- At least 70% time in target range of 63 to 140 mg/dL (3.5–7.8 mmol/L)
- Under 25% time above range
- Under 4% time below range
- Under 1% time below 54 mg/dL (3.0 mmol/L)

Adapted from Battelino T, Danne T, Bergenstal RM, et al. Clinical Targets for Continuous Glucose Monitoring Data Interpretation: Recommendations From the International Consensus on Time in Range. *Diabetes Care.* 2019;42(8):1593-1603.

group displayed lower glucose values in the morning and early evening than those in the SMBG group, thereby suggesting that postprandial hyperglycemia could be a key mechanism. The study also hypothesized that first trimester hyperglycemia, particularly daytime hyperglycemia, may contribute to LGA.

Recent commentary[17] based on data from CONCEPTT and Kristensen and colleagues[18] found that each 5% to 7% increment in psTIR in the second and third trimesters conferred lower odds of neonatal complications, namely LGA, neonatal hypoglycemia, and NICU admission. Such clinically significant implications also possessed potent economic ones; a secondary analysis[19] of CONCEPTT estimated that the total annual cost savings afforded by rtCGM use in pregnancy neared £10 million for England's National Health Service, the primary drivers of which were the reduced number and duration of NICU admissions.

Additional research is warranted to further define optimal targets for psTIR, psTAR, and psTBR. Similar efforts should be made to define targets for trimester-specific mean glucose, standard deviation, and coefficient of variation.

Self-Monitoring of Blood Glucose

Historically, frequent finger-stick glucose testing was the method of choice for glucose monitoring. While glycemic targets should always be tailored to individual risk of hypoglycemia, the target ranges[10] in **Box 3** are commonly employed for pregnant individuals with pre-existing diabetes or diabetes diagnosed during pregnancy. During a given day, for those not using CGM, SMBG should be completed while fasting in the morning, before and after each meal, and ideally at least once overnight.

INSULIN THERAPY IN PREGNANCY
Insulin Analogues in Pregnancy

Several insulin analogues have specific trials evaluating safety and benefit in pregnancy.[20–22] The rapid-acting analogues, insulin lispro and insulin aspart, display similar effects on metabolic control and pregnancy outcomes as human regular insulin[20–22] and accordingly are approved for use in pregnancy. One open-label, multicenter, randomized clinical trial[22] of 322 pregnant individuals with T1D concluded that insulin aspart was at least as effective and safe as regular human insulin and may confer additional benefit with respect to postprandial hyperglycemia and severe hypoglycemia. No formal trials have been performed for insulin glulisine. While no large trials have been conducted with the newer, ultrarapid-acting insulin analogues of aspart (Fiasp) and lispro (Lyumjev), these insulin formulations are generally regarded safe when used with a compatible delivery method. Inhaled insulin has not been studied in pregnancies complicated by T1D.

Long-acting analogues, insulin detemir and insulin glargine, demonstrate a lower risk of nocturnal hypoglycemia compared to neutral protamine Hagedorn (NPH), a

---

Box 3
Glycemic targets for self-monitoring of blood glucose

- Fasting: 70 to 95 mg/dL (3.9–5.3 mmol/L)

- One hour postprandial: 110 to 140 mg/dL (6.1–7.8 mmol/L)

- Two hour postprandial: 100 to 120 mg/dL (5.6–6.7 mmol/L)

Adapted from ElSayed NA, Aleppo G, Aroda VR, et al. 15. Management of Diabetes in Pregnancy: Standards of Care in Diabetes-2023. *Diabetes Care.* 2023;46(Suppl 1):S254-66.

difference due to improved variability in action profiles and duration of action.[20] Insulin detemir appears to have a slightly shorter duration of action (about 22 hours) and less variability in action profile than insulin glargine. A randomized controlled trial[23] of 310 women with T1D (79 of whom were randomized during early pregnancy) compared insulin detemir to NPH and found that insulin detemir conferred noninferior HbA1c and rates of hypoglycemia. Evidence for use of insulin glargine U100 and U300 is based on observational studies that have not documented safety concerns.[20,24] A recent open-label, international, randomized controlled trial[25] of 225 women compared insulin degludec with insulin detemir and showed similar pregnancy outcomes.

An important consideration with the long-acting insulin analogues is that their flat action profile may create challenges for individuals exhibiting dawn phenomenon. Solutions for MDI users could include the addition of a small, nighttime dose of NPH, or a small dose of a rapid-acting insulin analogue overnight or early in the morning.

Multiple Daily Injections of Insulin Versus Continuous Subcutaneous Insulin Infusion

Investigations comparing MDI to CSII have produced mixed results, partially due to variability in study design and outcomes. While the principal goal of CONCEPTT was to compare SMBG to SMBG with CGM, a prespecified secondary analysis[26] compared MDI to CSII in a nonrandomized manner. Women using CSII were less likely to smoke (9.6% vs 21.1%; $P = .019$) and more likely to be married or have a common-law partner (94.4% vs 81.3%; $P = .003$). Both groups had the same percentage of CGM users, and CGM compliance was similarly high (sensor use of 60% or more).

CSII use was linked to higher HbA1c at 24 weeks of gestation (6.37% [46 mmol/mol] vs 6.28% [45 mmol/mol]; adjusted $P = .014$) and at 34 weeks (6.54% [48 mmol/mol] vs 6.37% [46 mmol/mol]; adjusted $P = .001$). The frequencies of severe maternal hypoglycemia and DKA were similar between the 2 groups. psTBR was lower with CSII (3% vs 4%; $P = .03$). Obstetric outcomes were worse in the CSII group, as indicated by a higher percentage of hypertensive disorders (30.6% vs 15.5%; adjusted $P = .011$), particularly gestational hypertension (14.4% vs 5.2%; adjusted $P = .025$). Similarly, more infants of women who used CSII experienced NICU admission over 24 hours (44.5% vs 29.6%; adjusted $P = .02$) and neonatal hypoglycemia requiring intravenous dextrose (31.8 vs 19.1%; adjusted $P = .05$). There were no significant differences in preterm delivery, PE, cesarean delivery, birth weight, or LGA.

Two key limitations of this secondary analysis were the lack of randomization, as potential confounders included patient and provider preferences and expertise with CSII, and the absence of a prespecified protocol for insulin-delivery setting adjustments. The authors speculated whether women using MDI could have more aggressively adjusted insulin doses in response to gestational insulin resistance. The authors also questioned whether the complexity of prandial CSII settings (eg, extended bolus, dual or square wave patterns) may have hindered postprandial glycemic control, particularly in later trimesters. These points are salient when combined with the observations that insulin absorption is progressively prolonged with advancing gestation[4] and that there is increased daily variability in prandial insulin pharmacokinetics after the first trimester.[26] There were 25 people in the CSII group with low-glucose suspend features, but details about the use and frequency of insulin suspension could not be incorporated into the analyses.

A key strength of the secondary analysis of CONCEPTT was the ability to include participants who used CGM. While CGM use in pregnancy has been increasingly adopted in recent years, few other studies have compared MDI to CSII in people with T1D who concurrently used CGM. **Table 2** summarizes 2 useful studies[27,28] comparing MDI to CSII in individuals with T1D using SMBG.

Hybrid Closed-Loop Insulin Therapy

In the United States, no HCL system has an indication for use in pregnancies complicated by diabetes, and only one system currently has approval for use during pregnancy in the United Kingdom. As glycemic targets in currently commercially available HCL systems in the United States target a broader glycemic goal than the recommended gestational range of 65 to 140 mg/dL (3.5–7.8 mmol/L), current technology should be limited to select circumstances.

Many individuals who use commercially available HCL systems prior to conception may wish to discuss with their health care team continuation of use for prepregnancy preparation and while pregnant. Comprehensive discussion between people with T1D and providers experienced in HCL systems should be held prior to pregnancy. These

Table 2
Summary of select larger studies comparing multiple daily injections of insulin to continuous subcutaneous insulin infusion in self-monitoring of blood glucose users

Study	Mantaj et al,[28] 2019	Hauffe et al,[27] 2019
Size (N)	297	292
Design	• Poland • Single center • Retrospective (2010–2015) • No CGM	• Germany • Multicenter • Retrospective (2010–2017) • No CGM
Findings	• CSII had less postprandial hyperglycemia in second and third trimesters. • CSII had better fasting and nocturnal glycemic control. • Similar frequency of hypoglycemic episodes. • CSII has less risk of composite adverse neonatal outcome.	• CSII had more LGA. • CSII had similar pre-eclampsia, preterm delivery, neonatal hypoglycemia, cesarean delivery, NICU admission, and congenital malformations. • Similar HbA1c values prior to pregnancy and in each trimester.
Notes	• CSII group was more likely to have a planned pregnancy. • NICU-related outcomes were not examined.	• Glycemic control assessed only via HbA1c values; SMBG data not collected. • Individuals who switched from MDI to CSII in early pregnancy were included in the CSII group during the analysis. • Study methods did not describe formal pump training for those who transitioned to CSII. • Data did not align with prior observations that cigarette smoking increases LGA.

Abbreviations: CSII, continuous subcutaneous insulin infusion; HbAlc, hemoglobin A1c; LGA, large for gestational age; MDI, multiple daily injections of insulin; NICU, neonatal intensive care unit; SMBG, self-monitoring of blood glucose.

Adapted from Hauffe F, Schaefer-Graf UM, Fauzan R, et al. Higher rates of large-for-gestational-age newborns mediated by excess maternal weight gain in pregnancies with Type 1 diabetes and use of continuous subcutaneous insulin infusion vs multiple dose insulin injection. *Diabet Med.* 2019;36(2):158-166; and Mantaj U, Gutaj P, Ozegowska K, et al. Continuous subcutaneous insulin infusion reduces neonatal risk in pregnant women with type 1 diabetes mellitus. *Ginekol Pol.* 2019;90(3):154-160.

systems offer useful features to reduce hypoglycemia and hyperglycemia. Depending on the parameters of the specific HCL system, providers may ask pregnant individuals to enter "fake" carbohydrates or activate sleep mode to lower psTAR. Effective use requires the provider and patient to have a detailed understanding of which insulin pump parameters can be modified, and how the pump algorithm responds to predictions of hyperglycemia or hypoglycemia. Some individuals may achieve euglycemia by leveraging different modes of insulin delivery depending on the clinical scenario (eg, activating automated delivery only during the day or night).

Recent work on HCL systems with pregnancy-specific glycemic targets has demonstrated improvements in glycemic outcomes; however, further studies are needed to confirm improved maternal and neonatal outcomes. The largest trial to date occurred in the United Kingdom and was an open-label, multicenter, randomized controlled trial[29] of 124 patients that compared an HCL system using the Cambridge model predictive control algorithm (CamAPS FX) to standard of care (either MDI or CSII). The HCL system included the Dana Diabecare RS insulin pump (Sooil, Korea) and the Dexcom G6 rtCGM and targeted 100 mg/dL (5.5 mmol/L) in early pregnancy and lower values thereafter. Participants started their study intervention after the first trimester; both the intervention and control groups used CGM.

The HCL system was associated with higher overall psTIR (68.2% vs 55.6%), higher overnight psTIR (70.8% vs 56.7%), and lower psTAR (29.2% vs 41.4%). While psTBR and time below 54 mg/dL (3.0 mmol/L; termed TB54) were similar between the intervention and control groups, overnight psTBR was lower in the HCL system group (1.56% vs 2.57%). Closed-loop therapy was also linked to lower glycemic variability, as evidenced by lower standard deviation and coefficient of variation. While the trial lacked the statistical power to examine maternal and neonatal outcomes, the HCL system did not appear to increase the risk of maternal events such as hypoglycemia and DKA or neonatal complications such as hypoglycemia and NICU admission. Additional limitations of the trial included high racial homogeneity, the geographic concentration of study centers to the United Kingdom, and relatively high education status.

A small, multicenter, observational study[30] in the United States of 10 pregnant individuals using a noncommercially available HCL system provided additional support for the role of pregnancy-specific closed-loop therapy. The HCL system composed of a noncommercial, research-specific tandem pump (t:AP), an rtCGM, and a zone model predictive control-based algorithm designed for glycemic targets in pregnancy. The HCL system featured a daytime target of 80 to 110 mg/dL (4.4–6.1 mmol/L) and nighttime target of 80 to 100 mg/dL (4.4–5.6 mmol/L). The HCL system also automatically reduced meal boluses by 20% if the premeal glucose was below 70 mg/dL (3.9 mmol/L) and administered automatic correction boluses along with premeal boluses if the premeal glucose was above 100 mg/dL (5.6 mmol/L). In addition, insulin delivery was intensified if glucose values were rising when current values were in the range of 120 to 180 mg/dL (6.7–10 mmol/L).

Compared to the study run-in period—in which participants used their personal therapy and study-provided rtCGM—psTIR rose with closed-loop therapy (78.6% vs 64.5%; $P = .002$). Overnight psTIR was also higher with the HCL system (84.8% vs 61.3%; $P = .005$). psTAR was significantly lower with closed-loop therapy (19.7% vs 29.8%; $P = .033$), as were psTBR, TB54, and the number of hypoglycemic episodes per week (0.7 vs 4.0; $P < .001$). Nine of 10 participants achieved the guideline-recommended threshold of 70% in psTIR. There were no admissions for severe hypoglycemia or DKA. Owing to the study design, limitations included the absence of a control group and small sample size.

INTRAPARTUM GLYCEMIC MANAGEMENT

The goal range for intrapartum glucose of 70 to 126 mg/dL (3.9–7.0 mmol/L) seeks to avoid maternal hypoglycemia and curb maternal hyperglycemia, the latter of which promotes neonatal hyperinsulinemia and hypoglycemia after delivery. Uninterrupted insulin therapy is paramount to prevent DKA; dextrose-enriched intravenous fluids are administered concurrently as needed to prevent hypoglycemia. Insulin infusion with hourly finger-stick glucose monitoring is a safe and effective approach, but continuation of insulin pump therapy with frequent glucose monitoring can be considered in select individuals whose on-site clinical teams possess expertise in using these systems. Delivery of the neonate prompts transition of glycemic goals back to prepregnancy targets. As the placenta engenders progressive insulin resistance, delivery of the placenta prompts reduction of insulin doses at least by 50% to prevent hypoglycemia.

POSTPARTUM GLYCEMIC MANAGEMENT

Insulin requirements fall dramatically in the immediate postpartum period following the delivery of the placenta, and reductions of antepartum insulin regimens by 50% or more are often necessary. Breastfeeding can further increase the risk of hypoglycemia; an additional 20% reduction in insulin dose around the time of breastfeeding has been proposed to curb hypoglycemia.

The choice of agents included in the postpartum antihyperglycemic regimen depends on the mother's lactation status. Strategies to curb lactation-associated hypoglycemia include reducing basal rates prior to lactation in people using CSII and consuming a small amount of carbohydrates before breastfeeding in individuals on MDI.

A recent open-label, randomized control trial[31] of 18 individuals with T1D found that HCL system use conferred lower postpartum time below range (TBR) with unchanged TAR and TIR when compared to sensor-augmented pump therapy. Individuals who used closed-loop therapy exhibited less TBR (1.7% vs 5.5%; $P < .001$) and lower TB54 (0.3% vs 1.1%; $P = .008$). While these results are encouraging, more research remains necessary.

HEALTH CARE DISPARITIES IN CARE

Health care disparities significantly harm diabetes care in vulnerable populations. Social determinants of health (SDOH) such as race/ethnicity, socioeconomic status, and insurance status have been shown to worsen adoption rates of diabetes technology such as CGM and insulin pumps.[32] Concurrently, these SDOH are linked to worse glycemic control, as evidenced by higher HbA1c values and higher frequencies of DKA and severe hypoglycemia.[32] Multipronged approaches are necessary to address these issues and eliminate disparities in diabetes care and preconception care. Individuals who struggle to achieve optimal pregnancy-specific glycemic goals should be encouraged and supported with the knowledge that every 5% increase in psTIR is beneficial for the developing fetus.[17] Strategies to support all individuals with diabetes should include leveraging telemedicine to increase access to care by endocrinologists, lowering barriers to the prescription of diabetes technology by primary care providers, and systematizing the prescription of diabetes technology to mitigate implicit bias.

PRE-ECLAMPSIA PROPHYLAXIS WITH ASPIRIN

No large study has focused on the relationship between aspirin and PE in people with T1D. A recent multicenter, double-blind, placebo-controlled, randomized trial[33] evaluated 1776 women with singleton pregnancies at high risk for preterm PE. Of note, only 9 individuals with T1D were included in the study, which found that treatment with aspirin 150 mg daily reduced the risk of PE by 62%. A large, Danish prospective, observational cohort study[34] of 410 pregnant women with pregestational diabetes (257 individuals with T1D) examined the impact of aspirin prescribed at about 10 weeks of gestation. While there was no observed risk reduction for PE for participants with T1D, the study lacked a randomized design and may have possessed insufficient statistical power. Given the relative paucity of data, the current approach is that women with T1D who have other risk factors for PE should receive prophylactic aspirin, whose initiation should occur before 16 weeks of gestation.

SUMMARY

The care of pregnant individuals with T1D has experienced significant advancements in recent years. Preconception care has re-emerged as a core dimension of management. CGM plays an increasingly useful and beneficial role in gestational glycemic monitoring, a practice informed by improved maternofetal outcomes. While studies have not shown that CSII is superior to MDI for glycemic control, recent work has signaled that HCL systems with pregnancy-specific targets could meaningfully improve glycemic control and potentially ameliorate maternofetal outcomes while reducing self-care burden. Simultaneously, the rate of complications for pregnancies complicated by T1D remains suboptimal, which underscores the need for further research.

CLINICS CARE POINTS

- Pregnancies complicated by T1D display an increased risk of maternal complications (eg, severe hypoglycemia, PE, cesarean delivery) and neonatal adverse events (eg, perinatal mortality, congenital malformations, hypoglycemia requiring NICU admission).

- Gestational changes in insulin resistance confer an increased risk of hypoglycemia in the first trimester, and hyperglycemia in subsequent trimesters.

- Preconception care should ensure that individuals of reproductive potential understand glycemic and health goals prior to pregnancy and review schedules for the monitoring of retinopathy, kidney disease, and hypertension.

- CGM use in pregnancy, particularly rtCGM, improves glycemic control and maternal and neonatal outcomes while lowering self-care burden in a cost-saving manner.

- Further research on pregnancy-specific HCL systems is necessary; off-label use can be considered in select individuals and experienced providers after careful discussion of risks, benefits, and alternatives, as well as strategies to optimize pump use and algorithms.

DISCLOSURE

C.J. Levy has received research support from Insulet, United States, Abbott Diabetes, Tandem Diabetes, Mannkind, and Dexcom, United States paid to her institution, research supplies from Dexcom, and has received consulting fees from Dexcom and Eli Lilly.

REFERENCES

1. García-Patterson A, Gich I, Amini SB, et al. Insulin requirements throughout pregnancy in women with type 1 diabetes mellitus: three changes of direction. Diabetologia 2010;53(3):446–51.

2. O'Malley G, Ozaslan B, Levy CJ, et al. Longitudinal Observation of Insulin Use and Glucose Sensor Metrics in Pregnant Women with Type 1 Diabetes Using Continuous Glucose Monitors and Insulin Pumps: The LOIS-P Study. Diabetes Technol Therapeut 2021;23(12):807–17.

3. Kaur RJ, Smith BH, Ozaslan B, et al. Hypoglycemia in Prospective Multicenter Study of Pregnancies with Pre-Existing Type 1 Diabetes on Sensor-Augmented Pump Therapy: The LOIS-P Study. Diabetes Technol Therapeut 2022;24(8):544–55.

4. Murphy HR, Elleri D, Allen JM, et al. Pathophysiology of postprandial hyperglycaemia in women with type 1 diabetes during pregnancy. Diabetologia 2012; 55:282–93.

5. Benhalima K, Beunen K, Siegelaar SE, et al. Management of type 1 diabetes in pregnancy: update on lifestyle, pharmacological treatment, and novel technologies for achieving glycaemic targets [published correction appears in Lancet Diabetes Endocrinol. 2023 Oct;11(10):e12]. Lancet Diabetes Endocrinol 2023; 11(7):490–508.

6. Evers IM, de Valk HW, Visser GH. Risk of complications of pregnancy in women with type 1 diabetes: nationwide prospective study in the Netherlands. BMJ 2004; 328(7445):915.

7. Jensen DM, Damm P, Moelsted-Pedersen L, et al. Outcomes in type 1 diabetic pregnancies: a nationwide, population-based study. Diabetes Care 2004; 27(12):2819–23.

8. Lin SF, Kuo CF, Chiou MJ, et al. Maternal and fetal outcomes of pregnant women with type 1 diabetes, a national population study. Oncotarget 2017;8(46): 80679–87. Published 2017 Sep 16.

9. Dhanasekaran M, Mohan S, Erickson D, et al. Diabetic Ketoacidosis in Pregnancy: Clinical Risk Factors, Presentation, and Outcomes. J Clin Endocrinol Metab 2022;107:3137–43.

10. ElSayed NA, Aleppo G, Aroda VR, et al. Management of Diabetes in Pregnancy: Standards of Care in Diabetes-2023. Diabetes Care 2023;46(Suppl 1):S254–66.

11. Wahabi HA, Fayed A, Esmaeil S, et al. Systematic review and meta-analysis of the effectiveness of pre-pregnancy care for women with diabetes for improving maternal and perinatal outcomes. PLoS One 2020;15(8):e0237571.

12. Klein BE. Overview of epidemiologic studies of diabetic retinopathy. Ophthalmic Epidemiol 2007;14(4):179–83.

13. Ekbom P, Damm P, Feldt-Rasmussen B, et al. Pregnancy outcome in type 1 diabetic women with microalbuminuria. Diabetes Care 2001;24(10):1739–44.

14. Battelino T, Danne T, Bergenstal RM, et al. Clinical Targets for Continuous Glucose Monitoring Data Interpretation: Recommendations From the International Consensus on Time in Range. Diabetes Care 2019;42(8):1593–603.

15. Feig DS, Donovan LE, Corcoy R, et al. Continuous glucose monitoring in pregnant women with type 1 diabetes (CONCEPTT): a multicentre international randomized controlled trial [published correction appears in Lancet. 2017 Nov 25;390(10110):2346]. Lancet 2017;390(10110):2347–59.

16. Scott EM, Feig DS, Murphy HR, et al. CONCEPTT Collaborative Group. Continuous Glucose Monitoring in Pregnancy: Importance of Analyzing Temporal Profiles to Understand Clinical Outcomes. Diabetes Care 2020;43(6):1178–84.

17. Murphy HR. Continuous glucose monitoring targets in type 1 diabetes pregnancy: every 5% time in range matters. Diabetologia 2019;62(7):1123–8.

18. Kristensen K, Ögge LE, Sengpiel V, et al. Continuous glucose monitoring in pregnant women with type 1 diabetes: an observational cohort study of 186 pregnancies. Diabetologia 2019;62(7):1143–53.

19. Murphy HR, Feig DS, Sanchez JJ, et al. CONCEPTT Collaborative Group. Modelling potential cost savings from use of real-time continuous glucose monitoring in pregnant women with Type 1 diabetes. Diabet Med 2019;36(12):1652–8.
20. Mathieu C, Gillard P, Benhalima K. Insulin analogues in type 1 diabetes mellitus: getting better all the time. Nat Rev Endocrinol 2017;13(7):385–99.
21. González Blanco C, Chico Ballesteros A, Gich Saladich I, et al. Glycemic control and pregnancy outcomes in women with type 1 diabetes mellitus using lispro versus regular insulin: a systematic review and meta-analysis. Diabetes Technol Therapeut 2011;13(9):907–11.
22. Mathiesen ER, Kinsley B, Amiel SA, et al. Maternal glycemic control and hypoglycemia in type 1 diabetic pregnancy: a randomized trial of insulin aspart versus human insulin in 322 pregnant women. Diabetes Care 2007;30(4):771–6.
23. Mathiesen ER, Hod M, Ivanisevic M, et al. Maternal efficacy and safety outcomes in a randomized, controlled trial comparing insulin detemir with NPH insulin in 310 pregnant women with type 1 diabetes. Diabetes Care 2012;35(10):2012–7.
24. Di Cianni G, Torlone E, Lencioni C, et al. Perinatal outcomes associated with the use of glargine during pregnancy. Diabet Med 2008;25(8):993–6.
25. Mathiesen ER, Alibegovic AC, Corcoy R, et al. Insulin degludec versus insulin detemir, both in combination with insulin aspart, in the treatment of pregnant women with type 1 diabetes (EXPECT): an open-label, multinational, randomised, controlled, non-inferiority trial [published correction appears in Lancet Diabetes Endocrinol. 2023 May;11(5):e7] [published correction appears in Lancet Diabetes Endocrinol. 2023 Aug;11(8):e10]. Lancet Diabetes Endocrinol 2023;11(2):86–95.
26. Feig DS, Corcoy R, Donovan LE, et al. Pumps or Multiple Daily Injections in Pregnancy Involving Type 1 Diabetes: A Prespecified Analysis of the CONCEPTT Randomized Trial. Diabetes Care 2018;41(12):2471–9.
27. Hauffe F, Schaefer-Graf UM, Fauzan R, et al. Higher rates of large-for-gestational-age newborns mediated by excess maternal weight gain in pregnancies with Type 1 diabetes and use of continuous subcutaneous insulin infusion vs multiple dose insulin injection. Diabet Med 2019;36(2):158–66.
28. Mantaj U, Gutaj P, Ozegowska K, et al. Continuous subcutaneous insulin infusion reduces neonatal risk in pregnant women with type 1 diabetes mellitus. Ginekol Pol 2019;90(3):154–60.
29. Lee TTM, Collett C, Bergford S, et al. Automated Insulin Delivery in Women with Pregnancy Complicated by Type 1 Diabetes. N Engl J Med 2023;389(17):1566–78.
30. Levy CJ, Kudva YC, Ozaslan B, et al. At-Home Use of a Pregnancy-Specific Zone-MPC Closed-Loop System for Pregnancies Complicated by Type 1 Diabetes: A Single-Arm, Observational Multicenter Study. Diabetes Care 2023;46(7):1425–31.
31. Donovan LE, Feig DS, Lemieux P, et al. A Randomized Trial of Closed-Loop Insulin Delivery Postpartum in Type 1 Diabetes. Diabetes Care 2023;46(12):2258–66.
32. Majidi S, Ebekozien O, Noor N, et al. Inequities in health outcomes in children and adults with type 1 diabetes: data from the T1D exchange quality improvement collaborative. Clin Diabetes 2021;39(3):278–83.
33. Rolnik DL, Wright D, Poon LC, et al. Aspirin versus placebo in pregnancies at high risk for preterm preeclampsia. N Engl J Med 2017;377(7):613–22.
34. Do NC, Vestgaard M, Ásbjörnsdóttir B, et al. Unchanged prevalence of preeclampsia after implementation of prophylactic aspirin for all pregnant women with preexisting diabetes: a prospective cohort study. Diabetes Care 2021;dc211182.

Diagnosis and Treatment of Hyperglycemia in Pregnancy

Type 2 Diabetes Mellitus and Gestational Diabetes

Sneha Mohan, MBBS, Aoife M. Egan, MB, BCh, PhD*

KEYWORDS

- Gestational diabetes mellitus (GDM) • Pregnancy • Type 2 diabetes (T2DM) • Insulin
- Metformin

KEY POINTS

- The incidence of Type 2 diabetes mellitus (T2DM) in pregnancy and gestational diabetes mellitus (GDM) is rising globally due to a higher incidence of risk factors for metabolic disease.
- Screening for undiagnosed T2DM and GDM enables implementation of suitable management strategies to reduce maternal and neonatal complications.
- Insulin is recommended as primary therapy in T2DM and as first line in GDM when pharmacotherapy is indicated.
- Metformin can be used as adjuvant or alternate therapy.
- Multidisciplinary support during preconception, antenatal, and postpartum periods is essential for improving immediate and long-term outcomes.

INTRODUCTION

"Diabetes in pregnancy" encompasses pre-existing diabetes (including Type 1 and Type 2 diabetes mellitus (T2DM)) and gestational diabetes mellitus (GDM) (diabetes with onset during pregnancy and resolution after delivery).[1,2] Prevalence estimates of diabetes in pregnancy vary based on ethnic predisposition and differing diagnostic criteria. The US prevalence of GDM in 2021 was 8.3%.[3] Overall GDM rates rose by 27% in the United States between 2016 and 2021.[3] Prevalence of pre-existing T2DM rose from 0.42 to 0.78 per 100 deliveries between 1996 and 2014.[4] Increased

Division of Endocrinology, Diabetes and Metabolism, Department of Medicine, Mayo Clinic, 200 First Street Southwest, Rochester, MN 55905, USA
* Corresponding author. 200 First Street Southwest, Rochester, MN 55905.
E-mail address: Egan.Aoife@mayo.edu
Twitter: @SnehaMohanEndo (S.M.); @egan_am (A.M.E.)

Endocrinol Metab Clin N Am 53 (2024) 335–347
https://doi.org/10.1016/j.ecl.2024.05.011
0889-8529/24/© 2024 Elsevier Inc. All rights are reserved, including those for text and data mining, AI training, and similar technologies.

endo.theclinics.com

maternal obesity, older age at pregnancy, and physical inactivity among other risk factors (**Box 1**) contributed to these rate increases.[5]

In T2DM and GDM, there is a failure of the endocrine pancreas to accommodate and adapt to the metabolic stress of pregnancy, leading to varying degrees of hyperglycemia.[5] Infants of mothers with poorly controlled GDM and T2DM are more likely to be large for gestational age (LGA) due to fetal hyperinsulinemia.[6,7] This leads to increased risk of preterm delivery, prolonged labor, and the need for cesarean delivery in addition to neonatal respiratory distress syndrome, hypoglycemia, and electrolyte disturbances. Increased risk of gestational hypertension and pre-eclampsia add to maternal morbidity.[8,9]

Individuals with GDM have a 50% risk of developing GDM in future pregnancies[10] and a 10-fold increased risk of developing T2DM compared to those without GDM.[11] Offspring of individuals with GDM and T2DM have an elevated risk for childhood obesity, early development of insulin resistance, and subsequent T2DM.[12,13]

DIAGNOSIS
Pre-existing Type 2 Diabetes Mellitus

When T2DM is diagnosed prior to conception, additional diagnostic tests are not required during pregnancy.[1] In individuals with risk factors for T2DM, fasting glucose and hemoglobin A1c (HbA1c) should be tested at the first prenatal visit, ideally in the first trimester.[14] Universal testing can be considered, particularly in regions with a high background prevalence of T2DM.[14] Standard thresholds for diabetes diagnosis include fasting glucose $\geq$126 mg/dL, a 2-h post 75 g glucose load value $\geq$200 mg/dL, or HbA1c $\geq$6.5%.[2,15]

Gestational Diabetes Mellitus

There is heterogeneity in guidelines for GDM diagnosis.[16] The approach recommended by the World Health Organization,[17] European Board and College of Obstetrics and Gynecology,[18] and International Federation of Gynecology and Obstetrics[19] is a 1-step, 2-hour 75 g oral glucose tolerance test (OGTT) performed in all pregnant women between 24 and 28 weeks' gestation. Diagnosis of GDM is made if any of

---

Box 1
Risk factors for gestational diabetes mellitus

- Overweight or obese BMI
- GDM in a prior pregnancy
- Family history of diabetes
- Non-European ethnicity
- Polycystic ovarian syndrome
- Advanced maternal age
- Physical inactivity
- Multiple pregnancy
- Previous delivery of a macrosomic baby
- Previous stillbirth

GDM, gestational diabetes mellitus, BMI, body mass index

the glucose concentrations cross the specified cut-offs (**Table 1**).[5] These glycemic thresholds are based on results from the Hyperglycemia and Adverse Pregnancy Outcomes study which showed that women with glucose levels above these cut-offs had at least 1.75 times the estimated odds of adverse outcomes including birth weight, neonatal C-peptide, and body fat percentage greater than 90th percentile when compared to women with average glucose levels in this period of gestation.[8,14,20]

The American Diabetes Association (ADA) advises that either the aforementioned 1-step or a 2-step approach at 24 to 28 weeks' gestation may be used to diagnose GDM (see **Table 1**).[2] The 2-step approach involves an initial 50 g glucose challenge test performed non-fasting followed by a 3-hour, 100 g OGTT in those with glucose levels above a (variable) specified cut-off. Glycemic thresholds for the 3-h OGTT vary with the most common being the Carpenter and Coustan criteria (**Table 1**) which require 2 abnormal values to make a GDM diagnosis. The American College of Obstetrics and Gynecology supports the 2-step process described earlier adding that those with only 1 abnormal value on the 100 g 3-hour OGTT may also benefit from treatment, though further research is required.[21] Worldwide, various jurisdictions have modified the 1 and 2-step screening approaches to develop unique screening strategies.[22]

Two large trials recently compared the 1-step approach to 2-step testing and noted significantly higher rates of diagnosis of GDM with the former with no significant differences in maternal or neonatal outcomes.[23,24] While these studies lend support to the 2-step strategy, they do not address potential long-term benefits for identifying additional women at risk for T2DM.

Table 1
Strategies for screening and diagnosing gestational diabetes mellitus

	Oral Glucose Load, g	Glucose Cut-offs, mg/dL (mmol/L)	Number of Abnormal Values Required
One-step strategy			
2010 IADPSG/2013 WHO	75	Fasting ≥92 (5.1) 1-h ≥180 (10.0) 2-h ≥153 (8.5)	≥1
Two-step strategy: initial screening			
Non-fasting glucose challenge test	50	≥130,135 or 140 (7.2,7.5 or 7.8)	1
Confirmatory OGTT for positive glucose challenge test			
1. Carpenter and Coustan	100	Fasting ≥95 (5.3) 1-h ≥180 (10.0) 2-h ≥155 (8.6) 3-h ≥140 (7.8)	≥2
2. National Diabetes Data Group	100	Fasting ≥105 (5.3) 1-h ≥190 (10.6) 2-h ≥165 (9.2) 3-h ≥145 (8.0)	≥2
Modified testing strategy			
NICE guidelines	75	Fasting ≥(5.6) 2-h ≥(7.8)	≥1

Abbreviations: GDM, gestational diabetes mellitus; IADPSG, International Association of the Diabetes and Pregnancy Study Groups; NICE, National Institute for Health and Care Excellence; OGTT, oral glucose tolerance test; WHO, World Health Organization.

Interestingly, when different glycemic thresholds were compared in a recent trial, the use of lower cut-offs for the OGTT resulted in higher rates of diagnosis of GDM as expected but did not reduce the overall risk of LGA infants. However, when comparing the outcomes between women with milder GDM (diagnosed based on a lower OGTT cut-off) to their counterparts who were not treated (randomized to a higher cut-off), the risk of LGA was lower among those who were treated.[25] Overall, with lack of evidence to clearly support one approach over another, local policies for GDM diagnosis should consider availability of resources, background prevalence of T2DM, and risk factors for GDM to effectively identify women with the highest risk of complications.

Early Pregnancy Abnormal Glucose Metabolism

The timing of GDM screening is also called into question with the concern that 24 to 28 weeks' gestation is too late to prevent accelerated fetal growth which may begin as early at 15 weeks. However, early elevations in glucose levels are often no longer present by the time of routine OGTT which makes it difficult to identify at-risk individuals in early pregnancy.[26] A recent multicenter trial, showed modestly improved neonatal outcomes with GDM diagnosis and treatment less than 20 weeks' gestation, compared to women identified through conventional testing at 24 to 28 weeks.[27] The ADA recommends identifying those with early abnormal glucose metabolism before 15 weeks using fasting plasma glucose of 110 to 125 mg/dL or HbA1c 5.9% to 6.4%.[2] Nutrition counseling and weekly glucose testing is recommended for this group. Testing can intensify to daily, and treatment may be instituted if the fasting plasma glucose is predominantly greater than 110 mg/dL.[2]

MANAGEMENT
Preconception Care

For women with pre-existing T2DM in reproductive age, every clinical visit should address preconception counseling and pregnancy planning.[1] If pregnancy is not currently desired, long-acting reversible contraception (LARC) such as intrauterine devices, hormone implants, or injections should be recommended.[5] Women who are planning pregnancy should receive additional care including access to a multidisciplinary care team including an endocrinologist, maternal-fetal medicine specialist, dietician, and diabetes educator to optimize pre-pregnancy health.[15,28]

Periconception HbA1c <6.5% is associated with the lowest risk for congenital malformations, pre-eclampsia, and preterm birth.[29] Therefore, it is recommended to maintain HbA1c <6% if feasible while avoiding hypoglycemia. Achieving these targets is typically with use of insulin, as alternative glucose-lowering agents are not approved for pregnancy. However, metformin may be considered as an additive or alternative therapy.[1] Individuals should undergo a dilated eye examination within the year prior to pregnancy to screen and treat diabetic retinopathy which can worsen during pregnancy.[30] Kidney disease can increase risk for pre-eclampsia and preterm delivery and should be monitored. If the individual has end-stage renal disease, pregnancy should be deferred until after kidney transplantation.[31,32]

Comorbid conditions including hypertension and cardiac disease should be assessed and managed. Teratogenic medications including angiotensin converting enzyme inhibitors, angiotensin receptor blockers, and statins should be discontinued when the individual is ready to attempt pregnancy. Blood pressure should be tightly controlled and maintained at goal less than 135/85 with utilization of medications such as labetalol, nifedipine, or methyldopa.[5]

Folic acid supplementation is recommended for prevention of neural tube defects and should be initiated ideally at least 4 weeks before conception and continued at least until 12 weeks of gestation.[28]

Education on the changes expected during pregnancy including increasing insulin requirements, potential complications, and self-management of diabetes is essential. Lifestyle interventions including diet changes and physical activity to promote weight loss before conception and to ensure healthy weight gain during pregnancy are recommended.[1,15]

For women at risk for GDM (see **Box 1**), similar lifestyle interventions targeted at improving diet and promoting weight loss are recommended prior to conception. A meta-analysis analyzing lifestyle interventions showed a pooled reduction in risk of GDM by 18% with the benefits largely occurring when interventions are implemented before week 15.[33] However, it is challenging to implement these measures as a significant proportion of pregnancies are unplanned.[34]

Glycemic Targets and Glucose Monitoring

Women with pre-existing diabetes and GDM diagnosed during pregnancy require daily glucose monitoring.[1] Target glucose values for pregnancy are outlined in **Box 1; Table 2**.).[1] It is recommended to check glucose concentrations fasting, pre-meal, and 1-hour or 2-hour post-prandial.[35] While point of care capillary glucose testing is typically used, continuous glucose monitoring devices (CGM) have been approved for use during pregnancy and are increasingly employed.[36,37] However, there are no data to demonstrate that use of CGM in GDM/T2DM improves pregnancy outcomes. We additionally lack data to clearly define CGM time in range targets in this population.

HbA1c is unreliable for monitoring during pregnancy due to changes in red cell turnover leading to lower levels early in gestation.[38] However, the HbA1C goal in pregnancy is commonly accepted as less than 6% if this can be reached without significant hypoglycemia.[39] This goal may be relaxed to less than 7% in individual cases.[1]

Lifestyle measures

Lifestyle interventions focused on optimizing nutrition and physical activity are the cornerstone of managing GDM and T2DM in pregnancy as discussed later. A majority of pregnant women diagnosed with GDM can control hyperglycemia with lifestyle interventions alone.[1]

Medical Nutrition Therapy

An individualized nutrition plan which aligns with patient preferences should be created in coordination with a trained dietician. Excessive gestational weight gain is

Table 2 Glycemic targets during pregnancy	
Time	Recommended Glucose Levels; mg/dL (mmol/L)
Fasting	70 – 95 (3.9–5.3)
1-h postprandial	110 – 140 (6.1–7.8)
2-h postprandial	100 – 120 (5.6–6.7)

Adapted from American Diabetes Association—Standards of Care in Diabetes 2024

associated with worse outcomes and this should be avoided.[1] The Institute of Medicine has provided recommendations on appropriate weight gain during pregnancy (**Table 3**).[40]

The diet should focus on provision of adequate macro and micronutrients while avoiding significant postprandial hyperglycemia. While there is no evidence to suggest specific caloric intake during pregnancy, several trials utilizing low-glycemic diets, which on average contained about 1600 calories, showed benefit in reducing insulin requirements and led to lower birth weight when compared to control diets with higher glycemic index.[41]

The dietary reference intakes for pregnancy specify a minimum of 175 g of carbohydrates, 71 g of protein, and 28 g of fiber.[1,42] Polyunsaturated and monounsaturated fats should be prioritized and replace saturated and trans-fats.[1] The minimum carbohydrate recommendation is to avoid the risk of maternal ketonemia and ketonuria. Excessive fat intake can promote lipolysis and increase circulating free fatty acids which can unintentionally worsen maternal insulin resistance and should be avoided during pregnancy.[43]

Refined and processed sugars should be avoided. Whole grains, fresh vegetables, and some fruits should be substituted as ideal carbohydrate sources.[5] Carbohydrates can be limited to 35% to 45% of total calories consumed, distributed across 3 meals and 4 snacks throughout the day to minimize postprandial hyperglycemia.[44]

Physical Activity

Physical activity can reduce postprandial glucose excursions. A systematic review showed that physical activity interventions improved glucose control and reduced the need for insulin and insulin dosage when compared to controls.[45] However, the type of exercise varied across studies limiting evidence for a specific recommendation.[45] A general recommendation for 30 minutes of moderate-intensity physical activity (such as walking) at least 5 days a week should be made to improve overall outcomes.[21]

Pharmacotherapy

In individuals with GDM, intensification of therapy should be pursued within 1 to 2 weeks if glycemic targets are not met with lifestyle interventions (>15 to 20% of glucose values above goal).[1] In GDM, most guidelines recommend insulin as first-line pharmacotherapy.[1,21] Metformin and glyburide (glibenclamide) are also used to

Table 3
Institute of medicine guidelines for weight gain during pregnancy based on pre-pregnancy body mass index

Pre-pregnancy BMI Category	BMI kg/m^2	Recommended Total Weight Gain During Pregnancy, kg (lbs)	Recommended Weight Gain/week in Trimesters 2 and 3, kg (lbs)
Underweight	<18.5	12.5–18.0 (28–40)	0.44–0.58 (1–1.3)
Normal weight	18.5–24.9	11.5–16.0 (25–35)	0.35–0.50 (0.8–1)
Overweight	25.0–29.9	7.0–11.5 (15–25)	0.23–0.33 (0.5–0.7)
Obese	≥30.0	5.0–9.0 (11–20)	0.17–0.27 (0.4–0.6)

Abbreviation: IOM, institute of medicine; BMI, body mass index.
Institute of Medicine and National Research Council. 2009. Weight Gain During Pregnancy: Reexamining the Guidelines. https://doi.org/10.17226/12584. Reproduced with permission from the National Academy of Sciences, Courtesy of the National Academies Press, Washington, D.C.

treat GDM but are not FDA approved, and safety concerns exist.[1] Glucagon-like peptide-1 (GLP-1) receptor agonists, dipeptidyl peptidase-4 (DPP-4) inhibitors, and sodium/glucose cotransporter-2 (SGLT-2) inhibitors are not considered safe during pregnancy and are not recommended. Insulin remains the first-line agent for management of T2DM in pregnancy as alternate therapies are unlikely to overcome the level of insulin resistance encountered in pregnancy.[1]

Insulin

Twice or three times daily administration of neutral protamine Hagedorn (NPH) was traditionally used as a basal program during pregnancy, although recombinant insulins are now frequently used.[5,46] Insulin detemir is non-inferior to NPH and is associated with less hypoglycemia.[47] However, detemir is due to be removed from the US market in 2024. A recent trial compared degludec and detemir showing similar efficacy and safety outcomes in T1DM in pregnancy,[48] providing an alternative option to detemir. While there are no trials specifically evaluating glargine, it has been used extensively in clinical practice and observational data are reassuring.[49,50] Rapid-acting insulin lispro and aspart are effective to control mealtime glucose excursions. Typically, the starting total daily dose of insulin is 0.3 units/kg body weight.[46] It is reasonable to introduce basal and bolus insulin as required to target fasting and postprandial glucose values, respectively. Premixed insulin is not recommended in pregnancy as it is not possible to precisely refine the dosing of the prandial and basal components to achieve tight pregnancy glucose targets. In response to rapidly rising insulin resistance, frequent insulin dose adjustment is required, necessitating follow-up every 1 to 2 weeks with more frequent checks if control is suboptimal.[5] There are no data supporting use of insulin pumps in GDM/T2DM.

Metformin

When compared to insulin monotherapy, metformin shows similar glycemic control and is preferred by patients, but addition of insulin is frequently required.[51] Early initiation of metformin following GDM diagnosis shows it is noninferior to placebo with similar rates of insulin initiation while reducing occurrence of LGA infants and limiting maternal weight gain.[52] A recent trial assessed metformin added to insulin therapy in patients with T2DM or diabetes diagnosed in early pregnancy and showed no significant difference in a composite of neonatal outcomes but reduced the odds of delivering LGA babies compared to the placebo group.[53] A previous trial examining metformin use in pre-existing T2DM noted better glycemic control, lower HbA1c, and lower insulin requirements with metformin.[54] Mothers on metformin in this trial gained less weight and had fewer C-sections along with lower rates of delivering babies weighing greater than 97th centile for gestational age or greater than 4 kg. However, there were more babies born small for gestational age (SGA) suggesting that metformin should be avoided when intrauterine growth restriction is noted.[54]

Safety concerns remain as metformin crosses the placenta resulting in a high fetal-to-maternal ratio and increased risk for acidosis and placental insufficiency, possibly contributing to the increase in SGA babies observed in the aforementioned study.[54] Long-term data are limited but analysis of existing trial data shows that offspring of mothers with GDM managed with metformin initially have similar anthropometric measures but show significant differences when older, including higher weight, waist circumference, and waist-to-height ratio compared to offspring of mothers managed with insulin.[55]

Metformin is frequently used in women with polycystic ovarian syndrome to assist with fertility. While there have not been any significant adverse outcomes from studies evaluating this cohort, no benefit has been shown in preventing development of GDM, so the ADA does not recommend continuation beyond the first trimester in the absence of hyperglycemia.[1]

Overall, in the absence of more convincing evidence for efficacy and safety, metformin may be considered in GDM or T2DM after discussing risks and benefits, when maternal factors limit safe and effective utilization of insulin therapy.[1]

Sulfonylureas

Glyburide (Glibenclamide) has been studied in diabetes during pregnancy with evidence for good glycemic control.[56] However, glyburide crosses the placenta and promotes expression of placental glucose 1 transporter with concern for subsequent fetal overgrowth.[57] Glyburide use is associated with higher rates of macrosomia and neonatal hypoglycemia when compared to insulin or metformin therapy.[58] Long-term outcomes in offspring exposed to glyburide are unknown. Therefore, while it may be considered on an individual patient basis (eg, if insulin therapy is not affordable/feasible), it is no longer a favored choice for management of diabetes in pregnancy.[5]

Management of Maternal Complications

To prevent development of pre-eclampsia, guidelines recommend addition of low-dose aspirin (81 mg daily) after 12 weeks' gestation in individuals with pre-existing diabetes and after diagnosis of GDM if additional risk factors are noted such as chronic hypertension, autoimmune disease, obesity, age ≥35, or nulliparity.[1,59] In patients with microvascular and macrovascular diabetes complications, close subspeciality follow-up is required throughout pregnancy.

Diabetic ketoacidosis (DKA) can occur in any form of diabetes and is associated with significant fetal mortality.[60] Management is emergent and involves hydration, electrolyte management, and insulin therapy similar to management in nonpregnant individuals.[15,60]

Obstetric Care

Routine antenatal care should be completed per institute protocol with additional emphasis on comprehensive diabetes care. In individuals with pre-existing diabetes, a detailed fetal anatomy scan should be completed at 18 to 20 weeks' gestation with further evaluation as indicated.[15] After 32 weeks, all patients with diabetes in pregnancy should be closely followed up every 1 to 2 weeks including ultrasound evaluation of fetal wellbeing.[15]

Peripartum Care

In women with poor glycemic control, prior stillbirth, or diabetes-related obstetric complications, early induction of labor may be attempted between 36 0/7 and 37 6/7 weeks of gestation. Elective cesarean section may be considered when estimated fetal weight is over 4500 g. When antenatal steroid therapy is required, insulin may need to be added or increased to manage steroid-induced hyperglycemia for 3 to 5 days following administration.[15]

For patients with well-controlled pre-existing T2DM and GDM requiring pharmacotherapy, it is recommended to proceed with delivery between 39 0/7 and 39 6/7 weeks. If GDM is managed with lifestyle interventions alone, observation can occur for up to 40 6/7 weeks with appropriate monitoring.[15,21]

During labor and delivery, hourly glucose monitoring is recommended, and insulin is typically administered intravenously, although the subcutaneous route may also be utilized. A blood glucose goal between 70 and 126 mg/dL is advised.[5]

In women with GDM who were managed with lifestyle modifications in the antenatal period, hourly glucose monitoring is recommended with indication to start insulin if glucose is consistently greater than 100 to 126 mg/dL.[22]

Postpartum Care

Immediately following delivery of the placenta, women experience improvement in insulin sensitivity. In women with GDM, it is recommended to discontinue pharmacotherapy to avoid hypoglycemia.[21] In women with T2DM, insulin may be reduced by one-third to one-half of the pre-delivery doses with close monitoring for hypoglycemia.[15] While breastfeeding is strongly encouraged, glucose-lowering agents other than insulin and metformin are not considered safe for lactation.[15,21]

A neonatologist should oversee newborn care with close monitoring for hypoglycemia including a heel prick test to measure capillary blood glucose within 2 to 4 hours of birth. Breastfeeding should begin as soon as possible with supplemental formula as needed to prevent hypoglycemia. Tube-feeding or administration of intravenous dextrose is reserved for glucose levels that remain less than 36 mg/dL despite adequate feeding. The newborn is also at risk for hypocalcemia, hypomagnesemia, polycythemia, and hyperbilirubinemia and clinical monitoring is recommended.[5,22]

Women with GDM/T2DM should receive counseling on planning future pregnancies with discussion about LARC.[1] Women with GDM should undergo testing for undiagnosed pre-existing diabetes around 4 to 12 weeks' postpartum. The HbA1c in this period is unreliable and a 75 g OGTT with standard glycemic cut-offs is recommended.[1] Reports show that attendance for postpartum OGTT is as low as 5%; however, attempts to individually contact mothers through verbal and written communication may improve testing rates to 75%.[61]

Long-term follow-up is essential for women with a history of GDM due to their elevated risk for T2DM, stroke, and cardiovascular disease.[62] Testing every 1 to 3 years is recommended with the frequency varied based on prevailing risk factors. Fasting glucose, Hba1c, or a standard 75 g OGTT can be used to identify individuals who progress to T2DM.[1] Preventive strategies including lifestyle interventions and metformin may have benefit in preventing T2DM in women with history of GDM and prediabetes.[63] Further study is warranted to optimize care and prevent long-term complications.

SUMMARY

GDM and T2DM are common metabolic disorders of pregnancy. Early diagnosis and management by a multidisciplinary team is essential to prevent adverse maternal and fetal/neonatal outcomes.

CLINICS CARE POINTS

- Individuals with pre-existing T2DM should receive multi-disciplinary pre-pregnancy care to ensure optimization of diabetes control and related comorbidities prior to pregnancy.
- Diagnosis of GDM is via second trimester OGTT, though the precise strategy differs across guidelines.
- Lifestyle modification forms the cornerstone of GDM management.

> - Insulin is preferred pharmacotherapy for GDM/T2DM, with metformin as adjuvant or alternate therapy.
> - Postpartum care with long-term follow-up is required for early diagnosis of T2DM in women with GDM.

DISCLOSURES

Dr A.M. Egan is supported by a grant from the National Institutes of Health, United States: K23 DK134767.

REFERENCES

1. Committee ADAPP. 15. Management of Diabetes in Pregnancy: Standards of Care in Diabetes—2024. Diabetes Care 2023;47(Supplement_1):S282–94.
2. Committee ADAPP. 2. Diagnosis and Classification of Diabetes: Standards of Care in Diabetes—2024. Diabetes Care 2023;47(Supplement_1):S20–42.
3. Gregory E.C.W., Ely D.M., Trends and characteristics in prepregnancy diabetes: United States, 2016–2021. National Vital Statistics Reports; vol 72 no 6. National Center for Health Statistics; Hyattsville, MD, 2023.
4. Peng TY, Ehrlich SF, Crites Y, et al. Trends and racial and ethnic disparities in the prevalence of pregestational type 1 and type 2 diabetes in Northern California: 1996-2014. Am J Obstet Gynecol 2017;216(2):177.e171–8.
5. Egan AM, Dow ML, Vella A. A Review of the Pathophysiology and Management of Diabetes in Pregnancy. Mayo Clin Proc 2020;95(12):2734–46.
6. Desoye G, Nolan CJ. The fetal glucose steal: an underappreciated phenomenon in diabetic pregnancy. Diabetologia 2016;59(6):1089–94.
7. Pedersen J. Diabetes and pregnancy: blood sugar of newborn infants (Ph. D. Thesis. Copenhagen: Danish Science Press; 1952.
8. Lowe LP, Metzger BE, Dyer AR, et al. Hyperglycemia and Adverse Pregnancy Outcome (HAPO) Study: associations of maternal A1C and glucose with pregnancy outcomes. Diabetes Care 2012;35(3):574–80.
9. O'Sullivan EP, Avalos G, O'Reilly M, et al. Atlantic Diabetes in Pregnancy (DIP): the prevalence and outcomes of gestational diabetes mellitus using new diagnostic criteria. Diabetologia 2011;54(7):1670–5.
10. Egan AM, Enninga EAL, Alrahmani L, et al. Recurrent Gestational Diabetes Mellitus: A Narrative Review and Single-Center Experience. J Clin Med 2021;10(4).
11. Vounzoulaki E, Khunti K, Abner SC, et al. Progression to type 2 diabetes in women with a known history of gestational diabetes: systematic review and meta-analysis. BMJ 2020;369:m1361.
12. Lowe WL Jr, Scholtens DM, Lowe LP, et al. Association of gestational diabetes with maternal disorders of glucose metabolism and childhood adiposity. JAMA 2018;320(10):1005–16.
13. Scholtens DM, Kuang A, Lowe LP, et al. Hyperglycemia and adverse pregnancy outcome follow-up study (HAPO FUS): Maternal Glycemia and Childhood Glucose Metabolism. Diabetes Care 2019;42(3):381–92.
14. Metzger BE, Gabbe SG, Persson B, et al. International association of diabetes and pregnancy study groups recommendations on the diagnosis and classification of hyperglycemia in pregnancy. Diabetes Care 2010;33(3):676–82.
15. ACOG Practice Bulletin No. 201 Summary: Pregestational Diabetes Mellitus. Obstet Gynecol 2018;132(6):1514–6.

16. Bogdanet D, O'Shea P, Lyons C, et al. The oral glucose tolerance test-is it time for a change?-a literature review with an emphasis on pregnancy. J Clin Med 2020;9(11).

17. Diagnostic criteria and classification of hyperglycaemia first detected in pregnancy: a World Health Organization Guideline. Diabetes Res Clin Pract 2014; 103(3):341–63.

18. Benhalima K, Mathieu C, Damm P, et al. A proposal for the use of uniform diagnostic criteria for gestational diabetes in Europe: an opinion paper by the European Board & College of Obstetrics and Gynaecology (EBCOG). Diabetologia 2015;58(7):1422–9.

19. Hod M, Kapur A, Sacks DA, et al. The International Federation of Gynecology and Obstetrics (FIGO) Initiative on gestational diabetes mellitus: A pragmatic guide for diagnosis, management, and care. Int J Gynaecol Obstet 2015;131(Suppl 3):S173–211.

20. Metzger BE, Lowe LP, Dyer AR, et al. Hyperglycemia and adverse pregnancy outcomes. N Engl J Med 2008;358(19):1991–2002.

21. ACOG Practice Bulletin No. 190 Summary: Gestational Diabetes Mellitus. Obstet Gynecol 2018;131(2):406–8.

22. Diabetes in pregnancy: management from preconception to the postnatal period. National Institute for Health and Care Excellence (NICE); London, 2020. (NICE Guideline, No. 3.) Available at: https://www.ncbi.nlm.nih.gov/books/NBK555331/.

23. Hillier TA, Pedula KL, Ogasawara KK, et al. A pragmatic, randomized clinical trial of gestational diabetes screening. N Engl J Med 2021;384(10):895–904.

24. Davis EM, Abebe KZ, Simhan HN, et al. Perinatal outcomes of two screening strategies for gestational diabetes mellitus: a randomized controlled trial. Obstet Gynecol 2021;138(1):6–15.

25. Crowther CA, Samuel D, McCowan LME, et al. Lower versus higher glycemic criteria for diagnosis of gestational diabetes. N Engl J Med 2022;387(7):587–98.

26. Zhu W-w, Yang H-x, Wei Y-m, et al. Evaluation of the value of fasting plasma glucose in the first prenatal visit to diagnose gestational diabetes mellitus in China. Diabetes Care 2013;36(3):586–90.

27. Simmons D, Immanuel J, Hague WM, et al. Treatment of gestational diabetes mellitus diagnosed early in pregnancy. N Engl J Med 2023;388(23):2132–44.

28. ACOG Committee Opinion No. 762: Prepregnancy Counseling. Obstet Gynecol 2019;133(1):e78–89.

29. Jensen DM, Korsholm L, Ovesen P, et al. Peri-conceptional A1C and risk of serious adverse pregnancy outcome in 933 women with type 1 diabetes. Diabetes Care 2009;32(6):1046–8.

30. Egan AM, McVicker L, Heerey A, et al. Diabetic retinopathy in pregnancy: a population-based study of women with pregestational diabetes. J Diabetes Res 2015;2015:310239.

31. Ringholm L, Damm JA, Vestgaard M, et al. Diabetic nephropathy in women with preexisting diabetes: from pregnancy planning to breastfeeding. Curr Diab Rep 2016;16(2):12.

32. Tangren J, Nadel M, Hladunewich MA. Pregnancy and end-stage renal disease. Blood Purif 2018;45(1–3):194–200.

33. Song C, Li J, Leng J, et al. Lifestyle intervention can reduce the risk of gestational diabetes: a meta-analysis of randomized controlled trials. Obes Rev 2016;17(10): 960–9.

34. Moller AB, Petzold M, Chou D, et al. Early antenatal care visit: a systematic analysis of regional and global levels and trends of coverage from 1990 to 2013. Lancet Glob Health 2017;5(10):e977–83.

35. Metzger BE, Buchanan TA, Coustan DR, et al. Summary and recommendations of the Fifth International Workshop-Conference on Gestational Diabetes Mellitus. Diabetes Care 2007;30(Suppl 2):S251–60.

36. Yoo JH, Kim JH. The benefits of continuous glucose monitoring in pregnancy. Endocrinol Metab (Seoul) 2023;38(5):472–81.

37. Battelino T, Danne T, Bergenstal RM, et al. Clinical targets for continuous glucose monitoring data interpretation: recommendations from the international consensus on time in range. Diabetes Care 2019;42(8):1593–603.

38. Nielsen LR, Ekbom P, Damm P, et al. HbA1c levels are significantly lower in early and late pregnancy. Diabetes Care 2004;27(5):1200–1.

39. Abell SK, Boyle JA, de Courten B, et al. Impact of type 2 diabetes, obesity and glycaemic control on pregnancy outcomes. Aust N Z J Obstet Gynaecol 2017; 57(3):308–14.

40. Medicine Io, National Research Council Committee to Reexamine IOMPWG. The National Academies Collection: Reports funded by National Institutes of Health. In: Rasmussen KM, Yaktine AL, editors. Weight gain during pregnancy: Reexamining the guidelines. Washington (DC): National Academies Press (US) Copyright © 2009, National Academy of Sciences; 2009.

41. Viana LV, Gross JL, Azevedo MJ. Dietary intervention in patients with gestational diabetes mellitus: a systematic review and meta-analysis of randomized clinical trials on maternal and newborn outcomes. Diabetes Care 2014;37(12):3345–55.

42. *Dietary reference intakes: the essential Guide to nutrient requirements*. Washington DC: The National Academies Press; 2006.

43. Hernandez TL, Mande A, Barbour LA. Nutrition therapy within and beyond gestational diabetes. Diabetes Res Clin Pract 2018;145:39–50.

44. Blumer I, Hadar E, Hadden DR, et al. Diabetes and pregnancy: an endocrine society clinical practice guideline. J Clin Endocrinol Metab 2013;98(11):4227–49.

45. Laredo-Aguilera JA, Gallardo-Bravo M, Rabanales-Sotos JA, et al. Physical activity programs during pregnancy are effective for the control of gestational diabetes mellitus. Int J Environ Res Public Health 2020;17(17).

46. McIntyre HD, Catalano P, Zhang C, et al. Gestational diabetes mellitus. Nat Rev Dis Primers 2019;5(1):47.

47. Herrera KM, Rosenn BM, Foroutan J, et al. Randomized controlled trial of insulin detemir versus NPH for the treatment of pregnant women with diabetes. Am J Obstet Gynecol 2015;213(3). 426.e421-427.

48. Mathiesen ER, Alibegovic AC, Corcoy R, et al. Insulin degludec versus insulin detemir, both in combination with insulin aspart, in the treatment of pregnant women with type 1 diabetes (EXPECT): an open-label, multinational, randomised, controlled, non-inferiority trial. Lancet Diabetes Endocrinol 2023;11(2):86–95.

49. Mathiesen ER, Ali N, Alibegovic AC, et al. Risk of major congenital malformations or perinatal or neonatal death with insulin detemir versus other basal insulins in pregnant women with preexisting diabetes: the real-world EVOLVE Study. Diabetes Care 2021;44(9):2069–77.

50. Callesen NF, Damm J, Mathiesen JM, et al. Treatment with the long-acting insulin analogues detemir or glargine during pregnancy in women with type 1 diabetes: comparison of glycaemic control and pregnancy outcome. J Matern Fetal Neonatal Med 2013;26(6):588–92.

51. Rowan JA, Hague WM, Gao W, et al. Metformin versus insulin for the treatment of gestational diabetes. N Engl J Med 2008;358(19):2003–15.
52. Dunne F, Newman C, Alvarez-Iglesias A, et al. Early metformin in gestational diabetes: a randomized clinical trial. JAMA 2023;330(16):1547–56.
53. Boggess KA, Valint A, Refuerzo JS, et al. Metformin plus insulin for preexisting diabetes or gestational diabetes in early pregnancy: the MOMPOD randomized clinical trial. JAMA 2023;330(22):2182–90.
54. Feig DS, Donovan LE, Zinman B, et al. Metformin in women with type 2 diabetes in pregnancy (MiTy): a multicentre, international, randomised, placebo-controlled trial. Lancet Diabetes Endocrinol 2020;8(10):834–44.
55. Rowan JA, Rush EC, Obolonkin V, et al. Metformin in gestational diabetes: the offspring follow-up (MiG TOFU): Body composition at 2 years of age. Diabetes Care 2011;34(10):2279–84.
56. Langer O, Conway DL, Berkus MD, et al. A comparison of glyburide and insulin in women with gestational diabetes mellitus. N Engl J Med 2000;343(16):1134–8.
57. Wexler DJ, Powe CE, Barbour LA, et al. Research gaps in gestational diabetes mellitus: executive summary of a national institute of diabetes and digestive and kidney diseases workshop. Obstet Gynecol 2018;132(2):496–505.
58. Balsells M, García-Patterson A, Solà I, et al. Glibenclamide, metformin, and insulin for the treatment of gestational diabetes: a systematic review and meta-analysis. Bmj 2015;350:h102.
59. Henderson JT, Vesco KK, Senger CA, et al. Aspirin use to prevent preeclampsia and related morbidity and mortality: updated evidence report and systematic review for the US preventive services task force. JAMA 2021;326(12):1192–206.
60. Dhanasekaran M, Mohan S, Erickson D, et al. Diabetic ketoacidosis in pregnancy: clinical risk factors, presentation, and outcomes. J Clin Endocrinol Metab 2022;107(11):3137–43.
61. Carmody L, Egan AM, Dunne FP. Postpartum glucose testing for women with gestational diabetes mellitus: Improving regional recall rates. Diabetes Res Clin Pract 2015;108(3):e38–41.
62. Tobias DK, Stuart JJ, Li S, et al. Association of history of gestational diabetes with long-term cardiovascular disease risk in a large prospective cohort of US women. JAMA Intern Med 2017;177(12):1735–42.
63. Aroda VR, Christophi CA, Edelstein SL, et al. The effect of lifestyle intervention and metformin on preventing or delaying diabetes among women with and without gestational diabetes: the Diabetes Prevention Program outcomes study 10-year follow-up. J Clin Endocrinol Metab 2015;100(4):1646–53.

Evaluation and Management of Thyrotoxicosis During Pregnancy

Keerthana Haridas, MBBS[a,b], Tamlyn Sasaki, BS[c],
Angela M. Leung, MD, MSc[a,b],*

KEYWORDS

- Hyperthyroidism • Thyrotoxicosis • Thyroid • Pregnancy • Gestation

KEY POINTS

- Hyperthyroidism during pregnancy may appear similar to the biochemical and clinical physiologic thyroidal changes that accompany pregnancy, thus should be differentiated in order to guide the necessity of and type of treatments, if any are indicated.
- Medical management using anti-thyroid drugs is the mainstay of treatment of severe uncontrolled hyperthyroidism in pregnancy.
- Surgical management, if necessary, can be performed during pregnancy for the rare cases in which anti-thyroid drugs cannot be given and/or not tolerated for maternal Graves' disease or autonomous thyroid nodules. The risks and benefits of preoperative preparation with saturated solution of potassium iodide (SSKI) should be weighed in pregnancy.
- Radioactive isotopes, regardless if used for the diagnosis or treatment of thyrotoxicosis, are contraindicated in pregnancy, but can be considered in lactation under specific conditions and guidance.
- The optimal management of Graves' disease in pregnancy requires the multidisciplinary coordination between endocrinologists, maternal–fetal medicine specialists, neonatologists, and pediatricians for appropriate fetal surveillance.

[a] Division of Endocrinology, Diabetes and Metabolism, Department of Medicine, University of California Los Angeles David Geffen School of Medicine, Los Angeles, CA 90095, USA; [b] Division of Endocrinology, Diabetes and Metabolism, Department of Medicine, Veterans Affairs Greater Los Angeles Healthcare System, 11301 Wilshire Boulevard (111D), Los Angeles, CA 90073, USA; [c] University of Hawaii John A. Burns School of Medicine, 651 Ilalo Street, Medical Education Building, 3rd Floor, Honolulu, HI 96813, USA
* Corresponding author. Division of Endocrinology, Diabetes and Metabolism, Department of Medicine, Veterans Affairs Greater Los Angeles Healthcare System, 11301 Wilshire Boulevard (111D), Los Angeles, CA 90073.
E-mail address: amleung@mednet.ucla.edu
Twitter: @AngelaLeung9 (A.M.L.)

Endocrinol Metab Clin N Am 53 (2024) 349–361
https://doi.org/10.1016/j.ecl.2024.05.002
0889-8529/24/Published by Elsevier Inc.

INTRODUCTION

Thyroid hormone regulation within a narrow physiologic range is required for a healthy pregnancy, as well as fetal well-being. Uncontrolled hyperthyroidism poses risks to the mother, the delivery, and her infant, which can be mitigated by timely multi-disciplinary management. The presentation of maternal thyrotoxicosis during pregnancy requires the consideration of the various etiologies that produce similar clinical and biochemical findings, for appropriate monitoring and treatment as needed.

PHYSIOLOGIC ALTERATIONS UNDERLYING INCREASED THYROID HORMONE DEMANDS IN PREGNANCY

During pregnancy, the mother requires an increase in thyroid hormone production to ensure a sufficient supply for herself and the developing fetus.[1,2] Since the fetal thyroid does not produce its own thyroid hormone until 10 to 12 weeks of gestation, it relies on the placental transport of T4, particularly during early pregnancy for neurodevelopment.[3] The required increase of maternal thyroid hormone availability is achieved by several physiologic changes that occur during pregnancy (**Table 1**).

During pregnancy, increased estrogen stimulates the production of thyroxine-binding globulin (TBG) in the liver, particularly in early pregnancy when estrogen levels are high. Additionally, estrogen promotes the sialylation of TBG, decreasing its metabolic clearance rate. This effect of increased estrogen availability results in an approximate twofold increase in TBG levels during the first trimester, with a concomitant elevation in total serum thyroxine (T4) and triiodothyronine (T3) levels. Notably, the concentrations of free T4 and free T3 remain within their expected normal range during most of gestation.[2–5] Furthermore, human chorionic gonadotropin (hCG), secreted by placental trophoblasts, stimulates estrogen and progesterone synthesis in the corpus luteum during the first trimester of pregnancy. Due to its structural similarity to thyroid stimulating hormone (TSH), hCG also acts as a weak agonist of the TSH receptor to increase thyroid hormone production. This results in a transient increase in free T4 levels, which suppresses thyroid releasing hormone (TRH) activity and reduces TSH

Table 1 Reasons for increased maternal thyroid hormone requirements in pregnancy	
Physiologic Change of Pregnancy	**Effects on Thyroid Physiology and Serum Thyroid Function Tests**
Increased serum TBG concentrations	Increased total T3 and total T4 concentrations
Increased beta-hCG levels, particularly during first trimester	Stimulation of TSH receptor, leading to increased free T4 levels and decreased TSH levels
Placental D3 deiodination of T3 and T4	Decreased T3 and T4 concentrations, leading to increased T4 production
Increased GFR leading to increased renal iodine clearance; and transplacental passage of iodine to the fetus	Decreased maternal plasma iodine levels, leading to greater iodine requirements
Increased plasma volume and thyroid hormone distribution	Increased demand for higher maternal thyroid hormone concentrations

Abbreviations: D3, type 3 iodothyronine deiodinase; fT4, free thyroxine; GFR, glomerular filtration rate; hCG, human chorionic gonadotropin; T3, triiodothyronine; T4, thyroxine; TBG, thyroxine-binding globulin; TSH, thyroid stimulating hormone.

secretion. Serum hCG levels peak between 8 and 12 weeks of gestation, then reaching a plateau for the remainder of pregnancy.[2-4,6,7]

In addition, throughout pregnancy, type 3 iodothyronine deiodinase (D3) is highly expressed by the placenta, fetal epithelium, and maternal decidua.[8] D3 catalyzes the inner-ring deiodination of T4 and T3 to their biologically inactive forms, rT3 and 3,3'-diiodothyronine, respectively. This prevents excessive exposure of maternal thyroid hormone to the fetus yet stimulates an increased production of maternal T4 via feedback mechanisms.[3,9,10] Finally, there is an increase in renal glomerular filtration rate during pregnancy (resulting in increased iodide clearance) and loss of iodine transported through the placenta from the mother to the fetus, which necessitates increased maternal iodine levels during pregnancy. If this demand is not met by increased iodine intake, thyroid hormone production decreases, resulting in an increase in TSH secretion and possible formation of a goiter, including in the fetus.[2-4,8,11-21]

THYROID HORMONE EXCESS

The prevalence of hyperthyroidism in the general US population is approximately 1.3%, of which the vast majority ($\sim$70%) is biochemically subclinical disease. Common etiologies of hyperthyroidism include Graves' disease, toxic multinodular goiter (MNG), and toxic adenoma. Other causes of thyrotoxicosis (in which the cause of thyroid hormone excess could be extrathyroidal) include the use of certain medications (eg, amiodarone, lithium, multikinase inhibitors, and immune checkpoint inhibitors) or the presence of TSH-secreting pituitary adenomas, iodine-induced hyperthyroidism, subacute thyroiditis, Riedel's thyroiditis, choriocarcinomas, and ectopic thyroid-secreting tissues such as cases of struma ovarii. Individuals who ingest exogenous thyroid hormone (either intentionally or unintentionally) may also develop factitious thyrotoxicosis.[22] Worldwide, Graves' disease is the most common cause of hyperthyroidism, accounting for about 80% of cases. Uncontrolled hyperthyroidism is associated with complications such as atrial fibrillation, ischemic stroke, high output cardiac failure, osteoporosis, infertility, and increased mortality. Thyroid storm is the most extreme presentation of hyperthyroidism and can be life-threatening.[22]

OBSTETRIC AND OFFSPRING RISKS FROM UNTREATED MATERNAL HYPERTHYROIDISM

There are threats of uncontrolled maternal hyperthyroidism to the mother herself, the delivery, and the health of the fetus and newborn infant.[23-29] Maternal hyperthyroidism has been associated with an increased incidence of gestational hypertension and preeclampsia, which is thought to be mediated through increased sensitivity to adrenergic activity and increased activity of the renin–angiotensin–aldosterone system.[25,26,28-32] Uncontrolled hypertension, in turn, increases the risk of abruptio placentae, the premature separation of the placenta from the endometrium prior to the completion of the second stage of labor.[26,29] In addition, maternal hyperthyroidism, by causing insulin resistance and altering the cellular uptake of glucose, also increases the risks of developing gestational diabetes, which is ameliorated by correction of the hyperthyroidism.[26,28,29]

Thyroid storm and high output congestive heart failure are severe, life-threatening complications in pregnant women with overt hyperthyroidism.[33] Thyroid storm is usually precipitated in the setting of an infection, trauma, labor, or other surgery. It can be identified by the presence of hyperthermia, diaphoresis, tachycardia, widened pulse pressure, altered mental status, vomiting or diarrhea, and hepatic failure. While high output congestive heart failure may be observed in the setting of thyroid storm, it is also a separate entity resulting from the increased cardiac workload in the thyrotoxic state, physiologic cardiovascular changes in pregnancy and possible coexistent obstetric complications including gestational hypertension.[24]

Women with overt hyperthyroidism in the first trimester have a higher incidence of spontaneous miscarriages, especially those with positive thyroid antibodies, although the mechanism is unclear.[27,34] As pregnancy progresses, it has been observed that the mean gestational age of fetuses born to mothers with hyperthyroidism is lower than those born to euthyroid mothers, while controlling for age, alluding to a possible association with preterm births.[25,26,29–31,35] While the exact mechanism remains to be further elucidated, the possible binding of TSH to hCG receptors in the myometrium, stimulating uterine contractions, has been hypothesized.[35] Given that most subclinical hyperthyroidism in pregnancy is physiologic, an association with adverse pregnancy outcomes including miscarriages, preterm births, intrauterine deaths, or other adverse maternal or neonatal outcomes has not been shown with this more mild form of maternal hyperthyroidism.[23,30,33,35]

Maternal hyperthyroidism has been associated with a greater risk of fetal hyperthyroidism, characterized by tachycardia, growth retardation, accelerated bone maturation, and possible goiter,[36,37] particularly when maternal serum TSH receptor antibody (TRAb) concentrations are elevated to greater than three times the upper limit of the reference range.[1] Fetal hyperthyroidism develops as a result of stimulation of the fetal thyroid gland by the transplacental passage of maternal TRAb, even when mothers may be euthyroid.[1] Chronic TSH suppression in the fetus can also be complicated by fetal hypothyroidism after maternal TRAb levels have normalized.[37]

Maternal hyperthyroidism is also associated with neonatal complications including birth asphyxia, hypoglycemia, and neonatal jaundice.[28] Infants born to women with overt hyperthyroidism have lower birthweights than those born to euthyroid women, suggesting an association of thyroid hormone excess with intrauterine growth retardation (IUGR).[23,25,26,29–31] Growth restriction is likely related to elevated free thyroxine levels in the mother, which induce a catabolic state in the mother and the fetus as evidenced by increased protein and lipid degradation.[23] There is evidence that treatment and correction of hyperthyroidism, however, minimizes this complication.[27] Uncontrolled hyperthyroidism throughout the peripartum period has also been associated with intrauterine demise, regardless of whether maternal hyperthyroidism was diagnosed for the first time before, during, or in the 2 year period after pregnancy.[28]

SCREENING FOR THYROID DYSFUNCTION AND DIAGNOSING HYPERTHYROIDISM DURING PREGNANCY

Recommendations by the American Thyroid Association advise that a work-up should be performed either in patients with clinical evidence of thyroid dysfunction or with known prior thyroid disease.[1] In addition, women with high-risk features, including women aged 30 years or more and those with 2 or more previous pregnancies, prior preterm birth pregnancy loss, personal or family history of autoimmune disease, prior head and neck surgery, amiodarone or lithium use, recent exposure to iodinated contrast, or have body mass index 40 kg/m^2 or greater are advised to have TSH checked upon confirmation of pregnancy.

The interpretation of serum thyroid function tests in pregnant women requires several considerations related to the physiologic changes that occur during this life stage. In early pregnancy, the TSH level is inversely proportional to the level of beta-hCG. The normal range of TSH in pregnancy shifts downwards, with the largest shift occurring in the first trimester, starting in approximately week 7 of gestation, owing to the rapid rise in beta-hCG.[1] It should, however, be noted that about 10% of pregnant women without thyroid dysfunction can have TSH levels below the non-pregnant reference range, with about 5% of euthyroid women who normally have TSH levels less than 0.1 mU/L due to the suppressive effect of beta-hCG.[1,37] In addition, variations exist among different ethnic and racial groups, with less notable down-shifts of TSH levels observed in women of Asian descent.[1] While measurement of TSH is largely unaffected by the methodology used, the TSH multiple of medians (dividing the individual value by population median) can help decrease inter-assay variability.[1] Due to the effect of beta-hCG, the lower limit of the TSH reference range can be even lower in multiple gestation pregnancies.[4] Per guidelines by the American Thyroid Association and Endocrine Society, the TSH reference range in the first trimester is 0.1 to 2.5 mU/L (or a lower limit that is approximately 0.4 mU/L lower than that for non-pregnant individuals) and between 0.3 and 3.0 mU/L in the remaining trimesters when population-specific ranges, accounting for variations in race or ethnicity, cannot be used.[1,34]

In addition, due to an increase in circulating binding proteins during the second and third trimesters, some immunoassays may report lower free T3 and free T4 levels. More precise measurements of these levels using other techniques, such as equilibrium dialysis, ultrafiltration or liquid chromatography/tandem mass spectrometry, may not demonstrate these laboratory variations.[1,37] The latter techniques, however, are more expensive, time consuming, and less widely used.[1]

Serum total T4 and the calculated FT4 index are other options to monitor thyroid function during pregnancy; these levels increase through gestation weeks 7 to 18, reaching 150% of their pre-pregnancy levels and then plateau thereafter. Thus, a normal upper limit in pregnancy can be set by shifting their non-pregnant limits upwards by 50%.[1,37] Prior to this timepoint in the pregnancy, their upper limits can be calculated by adding 5% per week to the that of the pre-pregnancy reference range.

Thus, the diagnosis of hyperthyroidism is made by the simultaneous findings of a suppressed or undetectable TSH with elevated levels of either total T4, free T4, free T4 index, and/or free or total T3.[34]

The approach to the evaluation of thyrotoxicosis in pregnancy is outlined in **Fig. 1**.

DIFFERENTIAL DIAGNOSIS OF THYROTOXICOSIS IN PREGNANCY

Hyperthyroidism affects 0.1% to 0.4% of all pregnancies, with Grave's disease being the most common etiology (accounting for 95% of cases of overt hyperthyroidism). However, gestational transient thyrotoxicosis (GTT), the result of normal adaptive physiologic alterations of thyroid function tests during pregnancy, can closely mimic the clinical and biochemical presentations of hyperthyroidism among pregnant women. Less common causes of hyperthyroidism in pregnant women include toxic nodular goiter and hydatidiform mole.[1] The etiologies of hyperthyroidism in pregnant women should be differentiated to guide appropriate treatment.

The challenge with the diagnosis of thyrotoxicosis in pregnancy is to differentiate the clinical and biochemical features from a hyperthyroid etiology due to the normal physiologic changes that accompany pregnancy. Many symptoms suggestive of hyperthyroidism, including minor heat intolerance, intermittent palpitations, anxiety, and tremors, may be observed in a normal pregnancy. The diagnostic clues that distinguish pathologic hyperthyroidism from the normal adaptive changes of pregnancy (ie, GTT) are outlined in **Table 2**.

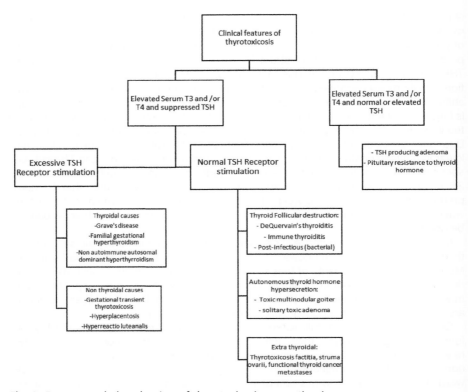

Fig. 1. Recommended evaluation of thyrotoxicosis presenting in pregnancy.

TREATMENT AND MONITORING OF GESTATIONAL TRANSIENT THYROTOXICOSIS

In those with abnormal thyroid function tests consistent with the diagnosis of GTT, treatment outside of supportive care is usually not required.[31] The symptoms of GTT can be managed by correction of dehydration and supportive control of vomiting. Serum thyroid function tests usually return to their reference ranges by 14 to 18 weeks of gestation.

TREATMENT AND MONITORING OF HYPERTHYROIDISM IN PREGNANCY
Management of Grave's Disease in Pregnancy

The recommended approach to the treatment and monitoring of Graves' disease in pregnancy is outlined in **Fig. 2.**

Medical management
Thionamides (propylthiouracil, methimazole, carbimazole) are antithyroid drugs that decrease thyroid hormone synthesis by inhibiting the organification of iodide and the coupling of monoiodotyrosine and diiodotyrosine. In high doses, propylthiouracil can also decrease the conversion of T4 to T3. Both methimazole and propylthiouracil are equally efficacious in the treatment of hyperthyroidism, cross the placenta resulting in equal concentrations in fetal serum, and alter fetal thyroid activity to the same extent. Propylthiouracil is dosed as 100 to 300 mg/day in divided doses every 8 hours. Methimazole is dosed as 5 to 30 mg/day and carbimazole as 10 to 40 mg/day, both in

Table 2
Distinguishing features of gestational transient thyrotoxicosis, Graves' disease, and autonomous thyroid nodules in pregnancy

	GTT	Graves' Disease	Autonomous Thyroid Nodule(s)
Characteristics	More likely with multiple gestation pregnancies	Both singleton and multiple gestation pregnancies	Both singleton and multiple gestation pregnancies
Symptoms	Hyperemesis more likely	Hyperemesis less likely	Hyperemesis less likely
	Palpitations rare or intermittent	Persistent palpitations	Persistent palpitations
	Weight gain throughout pregnancy (although weight loss may be seen if there is concurrent hyperemesis gravidarum)	Weight loss or inadequate weight gain throughout pregnancy	Weight loss or inadequate weight gain throughout pregnancy
	Nil-to-mild heat intolerance	+Heat intolerance and diaphoresis	+Heat intolerance and diaphoresis
Signs	Regular heart rate and rhythm	Tachycardia	Tachycardia
	Normal skin findings	Warm, moist skin	Warm, moist skin
	Normal reflexes	Hyperreflexia	Hyperreflexia
	Goiter absent	Goiter may be present with possible thrill and bruit	Goiter may be present with palpable nodule
	Normal eye findings	Possible thyroid eye disease	Normal eye findings
Investigations	Decreased/normal serum TSH	Decreased TSH	Decreased TSH
	Normal serum T3 and/or T4	Increased serum T3 and T4	Increased serum T3 and T4
	Negative serum TRAb titer	Usually positive serum TRAb titer	Negative serum TRAb titer

Abbreviations: GTT, gestational transient thyrotoxicosis; T3, triiodothyronine; T4, thyroxine; TRAb, thyrotropin receptor antibody; TSH, thyroid stimulating hormone.

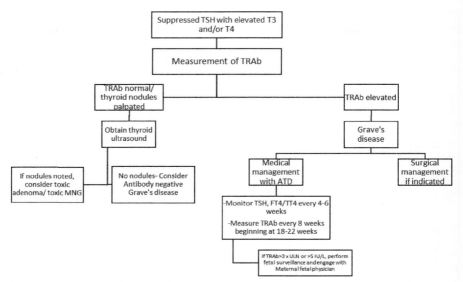

Fig. 2. Management of Graves' disease in pregnancy.

single daily doses due to their long half-lives. Adverse effects common to both classes of drugs include pruritic rash, gastrointestinal distress, and fever, reported in 5% to 10% of patients.[38] Serious reactions including ANCA vasculitis, agranulocytosis, and hepatotoxicity are rare but have been reported in pregnancy.[37] Agranulocytosis is reported in 0.3% to 3% of patients treated with methimazole, carbimazole, and propylthiouracil and is dose and duration dependent. Hepatotoxicity with propylthiouracil is generally hepatocellular and can be severe, with reports of some patients requiring liver transplantation and some instances of fatal hepatotoxicity. While on propylthiouracil, serum hepatic function tests must be monitored every 3 to 4 weeks to identify early hepatotoxicity.[31]

Both classes of drugs may also result in fetal anomalies. Use of methimazole and carbimazole during embryogenesis in pregnancy have been linked to a constellation of congenital anomalies in 2% to 4% of pregnancies. These include defects such as developmental delay, aplasia cutis, choanal atresia, tracheo-esophageal fistula, ventricular septal defects, omphalocele, athelia/hypothelia, and a distinctive facial phenotype characterized by scalp defects, slanted palpebral fissures, arched flared eyebrows, and a small nose with a broad bridge.[1,39,40] Use of propylthiouracil during organogenesis has also been associated with the development of cysts in the head and neck and urogenital anomalies, but the incidence is slightly lower than that of methimazole or carbimazole.

Although they are equally efficacious, to minimize the occurrence of maternal and fetal adverse effects, the American Thyroid Association, the Endocrine Society, and the U.S. Food and Drug Administration propose medical treatment with propylthiouracil in the first trimester and methimazole or carbimazole during the second and third trimesters.[1,31,37,38,41] A block-replace regimen (concurrent administration of levothyroxine and antithyroid drug) is not advisable due to higher doses of thionamides used in these regimens; because the placenta is more readily permeable to the thionamide than levothyroxine, the fetus would be predisposed to developing hypothyroidism.[42]

Beta blockers, when used for the symptomatic treatment of maternal hyperthyroidism, should be discontinued in 2 to 6 weeks, as longer durations of use have been associated with fetal bradycardia, IUGR, and neonatal hypoglycemia.[1]

During treatment or monitoring, thyroid function should be rechecked every 2 to 6 weeks, aiming for serum free T4 levels at the upper limit of the reference range as non-pregnant women or total T4 levels at 1.5 times the upper limit of the reference range for non-pregnant women.[37] TSH is a less preferred marker, as a normal TSH response can require weeks or longer to develop from the start of treatment, by which time fetal thyroid gland functioning may be suppressed. Suppressed TSH levels can thus represent the consequence of excessive antithyroid drug reaching the fetus. Once the above goal is achieved, the dose can either be maintained (with continued monitoring of thyroid function every 4–6 weeks) or cut by about 50% (with close monitoring of hormone levels every 2–4 weeks thereafter as long as TSH levels are within the reference range).[37]

Given the possibility of spontaneous remission of Graves' disease due to decreased autoimmunity during pregnancy, it is reasonable to withdraw medication in select patients, when pregnancy is detected and to repeat thyroid function testing within the first trimester.[43] It has also been noted that the dose of drugs required to maintain euthyroidism in pregnancy decreases as the pregnancy advances, and the antithyroid medication may even be discontinued in the second or third trimester.[37] The likelihood of disease remission in pregnancy is higher in those with disease duration less than 6 months, a normal TSH while on the antithyroid medication, whose thionamide dose requirements are less than 10 mg/day of methimazole or carbimazole or less than 200 mg/day of propylthiouracil, and those with low or undetectable levels of serum TRAb and without large goiters or orbitopathy.

Thyroid surgery

Thyroid surgery is considered in women with hyperthyroidism during pregnancy who have allergies or contraindications to the antithyroid drugs, in those non-adherent or unresponsive to medical therapy, or who require very high doses of thionamides (>30 mg/day of methimazole or carbimazole, or >1450 mg/day of propylthiouracil) to control the hyperthyroidism.[1,31] Surgery would also be recommended for patients with large compressive goiters that is producing urgent symptoms. Recent guidelines recommend that if surgery is advised in pregnancy, it can be safely done during any trimester.[44]

Following total thyroidectomy in women with Graves' disease, there is a slow, gradual decline in serum TRAb levels; thus, there remains a persistent risk of fetal hyperthyroidism, especially in women with a high concentration of TRAb (>5 IU/L).[45,46] In those intolerant of and/or unresponsive to medical therapy, the potential benefits and risks of preparation for surgery using beta blockers and a short course of potassium iodide solution should be discussed with the pregnant patient.[1]

Radioactive iodine

Radioactive iodide (RAI) therapy with I-131 is teratogenic and contraindicated in pregnancy, thus cannot be used for the treatment of Graves' disease during gestation.

Management of Other Causes of Hyperthyroidism in Pregnancy

Since RAI uptake scans cannot be performed in pregnancy, the diagnosis of autonomously functioning thyroid nodule(s) (ie, toxic adenoma or toxic MNG) cannot be made during gestation.

In women with autonomously functioning thyroid nodule(s), it is recommended to pursue definitive treatment of these conditions with thyroid surgery or RAI therapy, ideally to be completed at least 6 months prior to conception, to result in maternal euthyroidism and avoid exposure of RAI to the fetus once pregnancy is confirmed. If either of these options for definitive therapy is not achievable by the time of pregnancy, medical management may be carried out using antithyroid drug (ATDs) as outlined above. In severe cases of hyperthyroidism due to autonomously functioning thyroid nodule(s) that is unresponsive to pharmacotherapy, or in patients with compressive symptoms due to the condition, surgical management can be considered during pregnancy. RAI therapy with I-131 is teratogenic and contraindicated in pregnancy, thus cannot be used for the treatment of autonomous-functioning thyroid nodule(s) during gestation.

MONITORING AND TREATMENT OF FETAL GRAVES' DISEASE

Given the concern for fetal Graves' disease if maternal serum TRAb levels are greater than 3 times the upper limit of the normal range or greater than 5 IU/L at any point in pregnancy, fetal surveillance must be performed in conjunction with a maternal–fetal physician in appropriate patients with Graves' disease in pregnancy.[1,33] During the anatomy ultrasound done at approximately 20 weeks of gestation, the size of the fetal thyroid gland can be estimated to determine a potential diagnosis of fetal Graves' disease. In addition, any evidence of growth restriction or hydrops, oligohydramnios or polyhydramnios, advanced bone age, fetal tachycardia, and cardiac failure should be discerned.[31] Umbilical blood sampling is performed usually only if the diagnosis of fetal thyroid disease is equivocal using clinical, biochemical, and sonographic data.[31] In addition, all newborn infants should be screened for thyroid dysfunction between 2 and 5 days of birth.[1]

In the rare case of fetal hyperthyroidism, multidisciplinary care involving an endocrinologist, maternal–fetal medicine specialist, and neonatologist is crucial. Options for treatment in this complex scenario include antithyroid drugs administered to the mother and/or block-and-replace if the mother is treated for hypothyroidism as a consequence of previous pre-pregnancy radioactive iodine treatment or thyroid surgery.[1,37]

CLINICS CARE POINTS

- It is important to differentiate the etiology of hyperthyroidism in pregnant women, to guide appropriate monitoring and management during gestation.
- Medical management is the primary treatment of severe uncontrolled hyperthyroidism during pregnancy. Thyroid surgery may be needed in select cases. Radioactive iodine treatment is absolutely contraindicated in pregnancy.
- Multidisciplinary team-based care is essential in the setting of severe uncontrolled hyperthyroidism in pregnant women.

DISCLOSURES

The authors have nothing to disclose.

REFERENCES

1. Alexander EK, Pearce EN, Brent GA, et al. Guidelines of the American Thyroid Association for the Diagnosis and Management of Thyroid Disease During Pregnancy and the Postpartum. Thyroid® 2017;27(3):315–89.

2. Weeke J, Dybkjær L, Granlie K, et al. A longitudinal study of serum TSH, and total and free iodothyronines during normal pregnancy. Acta Endocrinol 1982;101(4): 531–7.

3. Soldin OP, Soldin D, Sastoque M. Gestation-specific thyroxine and thyroid stimulating hormone levels in the United States and Worldwide. Ther Drug Monit 2007; 29(5):553–9.

4. Kurioka H, Takahashi K, Miyazaki K. Maternal thyroid function during pregnancy and puerperal period. Endocr J 2005;52(5):587–91.

5. Glinoer D, Nayer PD, Bourdoux P, et al. Regulation of maternal thyroid during pregnancy. J Clin Endocrinol Metabol 1990;71(2):276–87.

6. Bernal J. Action of thyroid hormone in brain. J Endocrinol Invest 2002 Mar;25(3): 268–88. PMID: 11936472.

7. Ain KB, Mori Y, Refetoff S. Reduced clearance rate of thyroxine-binding globulin (TBG) with Increased Sialylation: A Mechanism for Estrogen-Induced Elevation of Serum TBG Concentration. J Clin Endocrinol Metabol 1987;65(4):689–96.

8. Huang SA, Dorfman DM, Genest DR, et al. Type 3 iodothyronine deiodinase is highly expressed in the human uteroplacental unit and in fetal epithelium. J Clin Endocrinol Metabol 2003;88(3):1384–8.

9. Soldin OP, Tractenberg RE, Hollowell JG, et al. Trimester-specific changes in maternal thyroid hormone, thyrotropin, and thyroglobulin concentrations during gestation: trends and associations across trimesters in iodine sufficiency. Thyroid 2004;14(12):1084–90.

10. Korevaar TIM, Steegers EAP, de Rijke YB, et al. Placental angiogenic factors are associated with maternal thyroid function and modify hCG-Mediated FT4 Stimulation. J Clin Endocrinol Metabol 2015;100(10):E1328–34.

11. Glinoer D, De Nayer Ph, Robyn C, et al. Serum levels of intact human chorionic gonadotropin (HCG) and its free a and β subunits, in relation to maternal thyroid stimulation during normal pregnancy. J Endocrinol Invest 1993;16(11):881–8.

12. Huang SA. Physiology and pathophysiology of type 3 deiodinase in humans. Thyroid 2005;15(8):875–81.

13. Taylor PN, Okosieme OE, Dayan CM, et al. Therapy of endocrine disease: impact of iodine supplementation in mild-to-moderate iodine deficiency: systematic review and meta-analysis. Eur J Endocrinol 2014;170(1):R1–15.

14. Glinoer D, De Nayer P, Delange F, et al. A randomized trial for the treatment of mild iodine deficiency during pregnancy: maternal and neonatal effects. J Clin Endocrinol Metabol 1995;80(1):258–69.

15. Dong AC, Stagnaro-Green A. Differences in diagnostic criteria mask the true prevalence of thyroid disease in pregnancy: a systematic review and meta-analysis. Thyroid® 2019;29(2):278–89.

16. Moreno-Reyes R, Glinoer D, Van Oyen H, et al. High prevalence of thyroid disorders in pregnant women in a mildly iodine-deficient country: a population-based study. J Clin Endocrinol Metab 2013;98(9):3694–701.

17. Sang Z, Wei W, Zhao N, et al. Thyroid dysfunction during late gestation is associated with excessive iodine intake in pregnant women. J Clin Endocrinol Metabol 2012;97(8):E1363–9.

18. Lambert-Messerlian G, McClain M, Haddow JE, et al. First- and second-trimester thyroid hormone reference data in pregnant women: a FaSTER (First- and Second-Trimester Evaluation of Risk for aneuploidy) Research Consortium study. Am J Obstet Gynecol 2008;199(1):62.e1–6.

19. Kostecka-Matyja M, Fedorowicz A, Bar-Andziak E, et al. Reference values for TSH and free thyroid hormones in healthy pregnant women in poland: a prospective, multicenter study. Eur Thyroid J 2017;6(2):82–8.
20. Hollowell JG, Staehling NW, Flanders WD, et al. Serum TSH, T4, and Thyroid Antibodies in the United States Population (1988 to 1994): National Health and Nutrition Examination Survey (NHANES III). J Clin Endocrinol Metabol 2002;87(2): 489–99.
21. Andersen SL, Olsen J, Carlé A, et al. Hyperthyroidism incidence fluctuates widely in and around pregnancy and is at variance with some other autoimmune diseases: a danish population-based study. J Clin Endocrinol Metabol 2015; 100(3):1164–71.
22. Leo SD, Lee SY, Braverman LE. Hyperthyroidism. Lancet 2016;388(10047): 906–18.
23. Chiu G, Zhang X, Zhao E, et al. Maternal thyroid disease and neonatal low birth weight: a systematic review and meta-analysis. Open J Obstet Gynecol 2017; 07(07):778–89.
24. Sheffield JS, Cunningham FG. Thyrotoxicosis and heart failure that complicate pregnancy. Am J Obstet Gynecol 2004 Jan;190(1):211–7. PMID: 14749662.
25. Millar LK, Wing DA, Leung AS, et al. Low birth weight and preeclampsia in pregnancies complicated by hyperthyroidism. Obstet Gynecol 1994;84:946–9.
26. Alves Junior JM, Bernardo WM, Ward LS, et al. Effect of hyperthyroidism control during pregnancy on maternal and fetal outcome: a systematic review and meta-analysis. Front Endocrinol 2022;13:800257.
27. Pillar N, Levy A, Holcberg G, et al. Pregnancy and perinatal outcome in women with hyperthyroidism. Int J Gynaecol Obstet 2010;108(1):61–4.
28. Sahu MT, Das V, Mittal S, et al. Overt and subclinical thyroid dysfunction among Indian pregnant women and its effect on maternal and fetal outcome. Arch Gynecol Obstet 2010;281:215–20.
29. Aggarawal N, Suri V, Singla R, et al. Pregnancy outcome in hyperthyroidism: a case control study. Gynecol Obstet Invest 2014;77(2):94–9.
30. Nazarpour S, Amiri M, Bidhendi Yarandi R, et al. Maternal subclinical hyperthyroidism and adverse pregnancy outcomes: a systematic review and meta-analysis of observational studies. Int J Endocrinol Metabol 2022 Jul 19;20(3): e120949. PMID: 36425270; PMCID: PMC9675093.
31. Luewan S, Chakkabut P, Tongsong T. Outcomes of pregnancy complicated with hyperthyroidism: a cohort study. Arch Gynecol Obstet 2011;283:243–7.
32. Osuna PM, Udovcic M, Sharma MD. Hyperthyroidism and the heart. Methodist Debakey Cardiovasc J 2017;13(2):60–3.
33. Moleti M, Di Mauro M, Sturniolo G, et al. Hyperthyroidism in the pregnant woman: Maternal and fetal aspects. J Clin Transl Endocrinol 2019;16:100190. Erratum in: J Clin Transl Endocrinol. 2020 Dec 17;23:100246. PMID: 31049292; PMCID: PMC6484219.
34. Leslie DG, Abalovich M, Alexander EK, et al. Management of thyroid dysfunction during pregnancy and postpartum: an endocrine society clinical practice guideline. J Clin Endocrinol Metabol 2012;97(8):2543–65.
35. Sheehan PM, Nankervis A, Araujo Junior E, et al. Maternal thyroid disease and preterm birth: systematic review and meta-analysis. J Clin Endocrinol Metab 2015;100(11):4325–31.
36. Glinoer D. Thyroid hyperfunction during pregnancy. Thyroid 1998;8(9):859–64.
37. Cooper DS, Laurberg P. Hyperthyroidism in pregnancy. Lancet Diabetes Endocrinol 2013;1(3):238–49.

38. Cooper DS. Antithyroid drugs. N Engl J Med 2005;352:905–17.
39. Taylor PN, Vaidya B. Side effects of anti-thyroid drugs and their impact on the choice of treatment for thyrotoxicosis in pregnancy. Eur Thyroid J 2012;1:176–85.
40. Valdez RM, Barbero PM, Liascovich RC, et al. Methimazole embryopathy: a contribution to defining the phenotype. Reprod Toxicol 2007;23(2):253.
41. Momotani N, Ito K, Hamada N, et al. Maternal hyperthyroidism and congenital malformation in the offspring. Clin Endocrinol 1984 Jun;20(6):695–700.
42. R- Abraham P, Avenell A, McGeoch SC, et al. 2010 Antithyroid drug regimen for treating Graves' hyperthyroidism. Cochrane Database Syst Rev 2010;20(1): CD003420.
43. S - Piccinni MP, Lombardelli L, Logiodice F, et al. How pregnancy can affect auto-immune diseases progression? Clin Mol Allergy 2016;14:11. PMID: 27651750; PMCID: PMC5025626.
44. ACOG Committee Opinion No. 775. Nonobstetric Surgery During Pregnancy. Obstet Gynecol 2019;133(4):e285–6.
45. Léger J, Carel JC. Diagnosis and management of hyperthyroidism from prenatal life to adolescence. Best Pract Res Clin Endocrinol Metabol 2018;32(4):373–86. Epub 2018 Apr 5. PMID: 30086864.
46. Hudzik B, Zubelewicz-Szkodzinska B. Antithyroid drugs during breastfeeding. Clin Endocrinol 2016 Dec;85(6):827–30.

Subclinical Hypothyroidism and Thyroid Autoimmunity in Pregnancy: To Treat or Not to Treat

Spyridoula Maraka, MD, MS[a,b], Chrysoula Dosiou, MD, MS[c,*]

KEYWORDS

- Thyroid peroxidase antibody • Thyroglobulin antibody • Euthyroid • Hypothyroidism
- Pregnancy • Levothyroxine • Thyroid hormone replacement

KEY POINTS

- Subclinical hypothyroidism in pregnancy is associated with adverse maternal and offspring outcomes.
- Current evidence shows obstetrical benefits of levothyroxine treatment of pregnant women with a thyroid-stimulating hormone (TSH) level greater than 4 mU/L.
- Thyroid autoimmunity in women is common and independently associated with infertility and adverse obstetric outcomes.
- Women with thyroid autoimmunity are at risk of developing subclinical/overt hypothyroidism.
- Recent randomized controlled trials do not show obstetrical benefits of levothyroxine treatment of euthyroid women with thyroid autoimmunity during gestation. There are not enough data to determine whether treatment of women with TSH 2.5 to 4 mU/L and thyroid autoimmunity is beneficial or harmful overall or in specific subgroups of women.

INTRODUCTION

Subclinical hypothyroidism (SCH) in pregnancy is defined as the presence of an elevated maternal thyrotropin (thyroid-stimulating hormone [TSH]) concentration with a normal free thyroxine (FT4) concentration.[1] Guidelines recommend using assay-specific and trimester-specific reference ranges for TSH and FT4,[1] but their availability is currently unknown. If pregnancy-specific TSH reference ranges are not available, an

[a] Division of Endocrinology, Diabetes and Metabolism, Department of Internal Medicine, University of Askansas for Medical Sciences, 4301 West Markham Street, Slot 587, Little Rock, AR 72205, USA; [b] Section of Endocrinology, Medicine Service, Central Arkansas Veterans Healthcare System, Little Rock, AR, USA; [c] Division of Endocrinology, Department of Internal Medicine, Stanford University School of Medicine, Stanford, CA, USA
* Corresponding author. Division of Endocrinology, Department of Medicine, Stanford University School of Medicine, 300 Pasteur Drive, S025, Stanford, CA 94305.
E-mail address: cdosiou@stanford.edu

Endocrinol Metab Clin N Am 53 (2024) 363–376
https://doi.org/10.1016/j.ecl.2024.05.010
0889-8529/24/© 2024 Elsevier Inc. All rights reserved, including those for text and data mining, AI training, and similar technologies.
endo.theclinics.com

upper reference limit of 4.0 mU/L may be used.[1] Depending on the TSH cutoff, the prevalence of SCH in pregnancy varies significantly (1.2%–42.9%).[2] SCH has been associated with adverse maternal and offspring outcomes, but the effectiveness of levothyroxine (LT4) treatment to improve outcomes is not well established.[3]

Thyroid autoimmunity, defined as antibodies against thyroid peroxidase (TPOAb) or thyroglobulin (TGAb), affects approximately 11% of reproductive-age women.[4] In this discussion, we will not address autoimmunity against the TSH receptor, as the focus is on autoimmunity associated with hypothyroidism. Overall, 5% to 14% of women have TPOAb, 3% to 18% have TGAb,[5] while 10% have antibodies against both antigens.[6] Antibody positivity and titers are positively associated with TSH increase in pregnancy.[7] The risk of both overt hypothyroidism (OH) and SCH in pregnancy is highest in the presence of both autoantibodies (odds ratio [OR] 44.69 [95% confidence interval (CI) 23.47–85.10] for OH, OR 6.26 [95% CI 4.29–9.13] for SCH) and is highly associated with the antibody titer.[8] Thyroid autoimmunity has been independently associated with adverse pregnancy outcomes and the effectiveness of LT4 treatment has been studied in recent randomized controlled trials (RCTs).

This review discusses the best available evidence on the impact of SCH and thyroid autoimmunity on pregnancy and the effect of LT4 treatment.

DISCUSSION
Subclinical Hypothyroidism

Impact of subclinical hypothyroidism on maternal and offspring outcomes
Thyroid hormones regulate key metabolic and anabolic processes in both mother and fetus throughout pregnancy.[9,10] SCH has been associated inconsistently with an increase in the risk of adverse pregnancy and offspring outcomes in individual observational studies.[3] In a systematic review and meta-analysis of 18 cohort studies comparing approximately 4000 pregnant women with SCH to euthyroid women, women with SCH were more likely to have pregnancy loss, placental abruption, premature rupture of membranes, and neonatal death.[3] However, there were significant differences in how SCH was defined and the gestational age at thyroid function screening, which could significantly influence the results. Moreover, common limitations of observational studies include lack of sample representation (nonpopulation-based studies) and lack of adjustment for important confounders.[3] Recently, individualized participant data (IPD) meta-analyses of prospective cohorts of pregnant women have allowed to uniformly define thyroid dysfunction and perform rigorous statistical analyses, increasing our confidence in the estimate results.

An IPD meta-analysis of 19 prospective cohort studies including 47,045 pregnant women found that SCH was associated with preterm birth (absolute risk difference 1.4% [95% CI 0.0–3.2]; OR 1.29 [95% CI 1.01–1.64]), but not with very preterm birth (gestational age <32 weeks) compared with euthyroidism.[11] Sensitivity analysis showed that the association of SCH with preterm birth was no longer apparent after additional adjustment for TPOAb positivity, suggesting that it is the TPOAb positivity that underlies any associations of SCH with preterm birth. Another IPD meta-analysis of 19 prospective cohort studies showed that among 39,826 pregnant women, SCH was associated with a higher risk of preeclampsia (3.6% vs 2.1%; OR 1.53 [95% CI 1.09–2.15]) compared with euthyroidism.[12] In continuous analyses, both a higher and a lower TSH concentration were associated with a higher risk of preeclampsia. Given the absence of clinical trials on the effects of different TSH treatment targets on adverse pregnancy outcomes, these indirect data suggest that an optimal TSH target for treatment could be in the middle of the reference range and highlight the relevance of monitoring thyroid function during pregnancy in women treated with LT4 to avoid undertreatment or overtreatment. Both IPD meta-analyses were adjusted for important confounders (maternal age, body mass index [BMI], ethnicity, smoking, parity, gestational age at sampling, and fetal sex).[11,12] Moreover, an IPD meta-analysis of 20 prospective cohort studies including 48,145 mother–child pairs found that SCH was associated with a higher risk of small for gestational age compared with euthyroidism (absolute risk difference 2.4% [95% CI 0.4–4.8]; OR 1.24 [95% CI 1.04–1.48]) and lower mean birthweight (adjusted risk difference -38 g [95% CI −61 to −15]).[13] Analysis was adjusted for maternal age, BMI, ethnicity, smoking, parity, gestational age at sampling, fetal sex, and gestational age at birth. Interestingly, the authors found an inverse, dose–response relationship of maternal FT4 (even within the normal range) with birthweight, where higher FT4 concentration was associated with lower birthweight. This result also prompts for careful consideration of potential risks of LT4 therapy and overtreatment during pregnancy.

Finally, of special interest is the potential impact of SCH on the neurodevelopment of the offspring. An aggregate meta-analysis of 11 cohort studies showed that SCH was associated with higher risk for child intellectual impairment (OR 2.14 [95% CI 1.20–3.83]) compared with euthyroidism.[14] Another aggregate meta-analysis of 15 cohort studies found that SCH in pregnancy was significantly associated with lower score on mental developmental index (relative risk [RR] −6.08 [95% CI −9.57 to −2.58]) and psychomotor developmental index (RR −7.29 [95% CI −10.30 to −4.28]) of the offspring compared with euthyroid women's offspring at 12 to 30 months of age.[15] However, an IPD meta-analysis of 3 prospective population-based birth cohort studies including 9036 mother–child pairs showed that maternal TSH in early pregnancy was not independently associated with nonverbal intelligence quotient (IQ) at 5 to 8 years of age, verbal IQ at 1.5 to 8 years of age, or autistic traits at 5 to 8 years of age (adjusted for maternal age, educational level, ethnicity, parity, prepregnancy BMI, smoking, gestational age at sampling, and child sex).[16]

Effects of treatment on maternal and offspring outcomes

Although SCH has been associated with multiple adverse maternal and offspring outcomes, the important question is whether LT4 treatment is effective in reducing the risk for these adverse outcomes.

A prospective study comparing the ability of universal screening versus case-finding to detect thyroid dysfunction provided indirect evidence.[17] Based on the presence of risk factors for thyroid dysfunction, 4562 women were randomized by the 11th week of pregnancy to universal screening versus case-finding. Women in the universal screening arm were checked for thyroid dysfunction and started on LT4 therapy if they had TSH greater than 2.5 mU/L and were TPOAb+. In the case-finding arm, only high-risk women were checked, whereas the low-risk group had their stored serum analyzed at the end of pregnancy, resulting in 34 women with hypothyroidism remaining untreated. There was no significant difference between the composite endpoint of adverse obstetrical and neonatal outcomes in the universal screening vs the case-finding group. Considering only the cohorts of low-risk women, complications were less likely among women in the universal screening than those in the case-finding group (OR 0.43 [95% CI 0.26–0.70]), driven by the events that happened to the untreated patients with hypothyroidism.

Since then, multiple RCTs have assessed the effects of LT4 treatment on maternal and offspring outcomes (**Table 1**). In the controlled antenatal thyroid screening (CATS) study, 21,846 women were randomized at a median of 12 weeks 3 days of gestation to a group screened for thyroid dysfunction or to a control group who had their

Table 1
Summary of the outcomes from randomized controlled trials of levothyroxine treatment of subclinical hypothyroidism during pregnancy

Study Characteristics	Lazarus et al,[18] 2012[b]	Nazarpour et al,[22] 2017	Casey et al,[20] 2017	Nazarpour et al,[21] 2018	Hales et al,[19] 2018[b]	Nazarpour et al, 2023
Country	United Kingdom and Italy	Iran	United States	Iran	United Kingdom and Italy	Iran
LT4 group (N =)	186	56	339	183	63	189
Control group (N =)	197	58	338	183	51	168
Population	TSH >97.5th percentile FT4 ≥2.5 percentile	TSH 2.5–10 mU/L Normal FT4 index TPOAb⁺	TSH ≥4.0 mU/L Normal FT4	TSH 2.5–10 mU/L Normal FT4 index TPOAb⁻	TSH >97.5th percentile FT4 ≥2.5th percentile	TSH 2.5–10 mU/L Normal FT4 index
Maternal outcomes						
Pregnancy loss[a]	N/A	-	-	-	N/A	N/A
Preterm delivery	N/A	✓	-	✓[c]	N/A	N/A
Placental abruption	N/A	-	-	-	N/A	N/A
Gestational diabetes	N/A	N/A	-	N/A	N/A	N/A
Gestational hypertension	N/A	N/A	-	N/A	N/A	N/A
Preeclampsia	N/A	N/A	-	N/A	N/A	N/A
Neonatal/offspring outcomes						
Neonatal birth weight	N/A	-	-	-	N/A	N/A
Head circumference	N/A	-	-	-	N/A	N/A
Neonatal admission	N/A	✓	-	-	N/A	N/A
Apgar score	N/A	N/A	-	N/A	N/A	N/A
Neonatal death	N/A	N/A	-	N/A	N/A	N/A
Offspring IQ	-	N/A	-	N/A	-	N/A
Development/behavior	-	N/A	-	N/A	N/A	-

✓ Positive effect, - Neutral effect

Abbreviations: FT4, free thyroxine; LT4, levothyroxine; N/A, not assessed; SCH, subclinical hypothyroidism; TPOAb, thyroid peroxidase antibody; TSH, thyroid-stimulating hormone.

[a] Includes miscarriage and stillbirth.

[b] These studies investigated the effect of LT4 on pregnant women with TSH >97.5th percentile, FT4 <2.5th percentile, or both; we present the data on the subgroup with SCH.

stored serum analyzed at the end of pregnancy (untreated).[18] Treatment with 150 mcg of LT4 was started at a median of 13 weeks 3 days of gestation in screened women found to have a TSH level greater than 97.5th percentile, an FT4 level less than 2.5th percentile, or both. Treatment was adjusted to achieve a target TSH of 0.1 to 1.0 mU/L. There was no difference between groups in the IQ of children at 3 years of age (treated mean IQ 99 vs untreated mean IQ 100) and the percentage of children with IQ less than 85. A subgroup analysis including only women with SCH had similar results. Study limitations included the late initiation of LT4 therapy (possibly too late in gestation to have a major influence on brain development), the relatively high, fixed LT4 dosing that could have negatively impacted IQ, the questionable accuracy of IQ testing in 3 year old children, and inadequate power to detect subtle differences in cognition. Data from the CATS-II study showed that LT4 therapy did not improve child cognition at age 9.5 years, confirming long term the CATS study results.[19] In another multicenter RCT, pregnant women with SCH (TSH >4.0 mU/L, normal FT4 levels) were randomized to LT4 treatment versus placebo.[20] There was no benefit of LT4 treatment regarding offspring IQ at 5 years, selected adverse pregnancy outcomes (preterm delivery, gestational hypertension, preeclampsia, gestational diabetes, and placental abruption), and adverse neonatal outcomes (neonatal death, low Apgar score, admission to the neonatal intensive care unit, low birth weight, and congenital malformations). A post hoc analysis found no significant interaction according to TPOAb level. However, LT4 therapy was initiated at 17 weeks of gestation on average. Due to the late randomization, the study was not able to adequately assess the outcome of miscarriage. Another single-blinded RCT showed that there was no beneficial effect of LT4 therapy in reducing preterm delivery in SCH TPOAb$^-$ women with TSH of 2.5 to 10.0 mU/L.[21] However, a subgroup analysis showed that LT4 could decrease this complication using a TSH cutoff greater than 4.0 mU/L (RR 0.38 [95% CI 0.15–0.98]; P = .04). Similarly, the Tehran Thyroid and Pregnancy Study showed a 70% and 83% decrease in preterm delivery and neonatal hospital admissions, respectively, in LT4-treated pregnant women who were TPOAb$^+$ compared with untreated women (TSH 2.5–10.0 mU/L).[22] Subgroup analysis showed that the benefit of LT4 treatment was observed only among TPOAb$^+$ women with TSH greater than 4.0 mU/L. A follow-up of these trials showed that there was no difference in the neurodevelopmental score of offspring at 3 years in mothers with SCH randomized to LT4 treatment versus no treatment.[23]

With regard to pregnancy loss, the best available evidence is from a US national cohort study, which compared 843 pregnant women with SCH who received thyroid hormone treatment with 4562 women who remained untreated.[24] The study showed that LT4 therapy was not only associated with decreased risk of pregnancy loss (OR 0.45 [95% CI 0.30–0.65]) but also with higher risk of preterm delivery (OR 1.60 [95% CI 1.14–2.24]), gestational diabetes (OR 1.37 [95% CI 1.05–1.79]), and preeclampsia (OR 1.61 [95% CI 1.10–2.37]). A stratified analysis showed that the treated women with a higher TSH level (4.1–10 mU/L) were the ones who had the benefit of fewer pregnancy losses and not the ones with milder TSH elevation (2.5–4.0 mU/L). This lack of benefit together with the noted risk of adverse events raised the concern of possible overtreatment of women with TSH 2.5 to 4.0 mU/L. Study limitations included the retrospective observational design, the potential for misclassification of treatment and confounders, lack of data on gestational age at initiation of LT4 therapy and TPOAb status, and possible selection bias.

Thyroid Autoimmunity

Two significant physiologic events affect the phenotype of thyroid autoimmunity during pregnancy. First, the pregnant state poses a "stress test" for the thyroid, due to a number of changes that cause an increased demand for thyroid hormone by up to 50% by midgestation.[25] Women who are already on thyroid hormone prepregnancy need to therefore increase their dose,[26–28] while euthyroid women with autoimmunity have a 16% to 19% risk of developing hypothyroidism.[6,29] Higher baseline TSH and TPOAb titers are associated with greater risk.[6] Second, progesterone induces a state of immunotolerance, shifting the immune response from a Th1 to a more dominant Th2 profile, while increasing the population of regulatory T cells.[30] Consequently, thyroid antibody titers decrease during gestation,[31] by an average of 60%.[6,29] The reverse happens in the postpartum phase, where the sudden drop in progesterone results in flares of autoimmune disease, manifesting as postpartum thyroiditis in 50% of women.[32,33] These changes influence disease presentation as well as the levels of thyroid autoantibodies.

Impact of thyroid autoimmunity on obstetrical outcomes and potential mechanisms
Thyroid autoimmunity is independently associated with an increased risk of infertility,[34] low ovarian reserve,[35,36] and lower live birth rates,[37] as well as obstetrical and fetal complications, even in the absence of overt thyroid dysfunction. In a landmark article in 1990, Stagnaro-Green and colleagues first described the association of thyroid autoimmunity with spontaneous miscarriage.[38] Meta-analyses of more than 10 cohort studies have confirmed a 2 to 4 fold increase in risk of mostly first trimester miscarriage in the presence of thyroid autoimmunity.[39,40] The effect of autoimmunity appears to be additive to that of TSH elevation alone.[41] Thyroid autoimmunity is also associated with an increased risk for recurrent miscarriages,[42] 4 fold increase in the incidence of placental abruption,[43] and an increased risk of preterm birth.[11,39,41] Traditionally, these risks have been predominantly thought to be due to a relative thyroid hormone insufficiency at the level of the placental-fetal unit, due to limited thyroidal reserve. This possibility was supported by the observation that supplementation with thyroid hormone improved obstetric outcomes in initial RCTs[17,29] as well as the fact that TPOAb positivity blunts the normal thyroidal response to human chorionic gonadotropin (HCG).[44] Alternatively, the antibodies themselves may be directly pathogenic to ovarian antigens[45] or be a marker of more generalized autoimmunity that adversely affects pregnancy success.[46] The antibodies may also directly affect oocyte health, as studies of women undergoing assisted reproductive technology (ART) have shown that the quality of the embryos obtained from oocytes of TPOAb+ women is inferior to that obtained from TPOAb− women.[47]

Effects of treatment on obstetrical outcomes
Prior to the latest American Thyroid Association (ATA) clinical guidelines for the management of thyroid disease in pregnancy,[1] 2 RCTs from Italy investigated the effect of LT4 on obstetrical outcomes in euthyroid women with thyroid autoimmunity. A 2006 RCT of 115 TPOAb+ euthyroid patients (TSH <4.2 mU/L) showed a beneficial effect of LT4 treatment on reducing miscarriage rates from 13.8% to 3.5% and preterm delivery rates from 22.4% to 7%.[29] A follow-up RCT study of 393 women with thyroid autoimmunity and a TSH less than 2.5 mU/L, showed that LT4 had no effect on miscarriage or preterm delivery rates.[48] A limitation of the second study was that 49% of women in the control group were also treated with LT4 starting in the second or third trimester (per protocol design, treatment was initiated if TSH rose to >3 mU/L); this could have skewed results toward the null hypothesis.

Since 2017, 3 large RCTs have failed to show an obstetrical benefit of LT4 supplementation in euthyroid patients with thyroid autoimmunity (POSTAL,[49] TABLET,[50] and T4LIFE[51]; **Table 2**). The TABLET trial showed that 952 women with a history of

Table 2
Randomized controlled trials of levothyroxine impact on obstetrical outcomes in euthyroid women with thyroid autoimmunity

Trial, Year	Negro et al,[29] 2006[a]	Negro et al,[48] 2016	POSTAL,[49] 2017	TABLET,[50] 2019[c]	T4LIFE,[51] 2022[d]
Location	Italy	Italy	China	United Kingdom	Netherlands, Belgium, and Denmark
N	115	393	600	952	187[e]
Population	All pregnant women, TPOAb >100 kIU/L, TSH 0.27–4.2 mU/L, control = no treatment	All pregnant women, TPOAb >16 IU/mL TSH 0.5–2.5 mU/L, control = no treatment[b]	Undergoing IVF, excluded RPL, TPOAb >60 IU/mL, TSH 0.5–4.78 mU/L, control = no treatment	h/o miscarriage or infertility, conceiving naturally or with ART, TPOAb greater than individual laboratory thresholds, TSH 0.44–3.63 mU/L, control = placebo	h/o RPL, conceiving both naturally and with ART, TPOAb greater than individual laboratory thresholds, TSH within individual laboratory ref range, control = placebo
Clinical pregnancy (%)					
Control	NA	NA	37.7	58.3	78
LT4	NA	NA	35.7	56.6	73
Miscarriage (%)					
Control	13.8	14.9	10.6	29.6	33
LT4	3.5*	11.6	10.3	28.2	23
Live birth (%)					
Control	NA	NA	32.3	37.9	48
LT4	NA	NA	31.7	37.4	50
Preterm delivery (%)					
Control	22.4	10.8	19.6	NA	4
LT4	7.0*	6.9	22.1	NA	6

(continued on next page)

Table 2
(continued)

Trial, Year	Negro et al,[29] 2006[a]	Negro et al,[48] 2016	POSTAL,[49] 2017	TABLET,[50] 2019[c]	T4LIFE,[51] 2022[d]
TSH, prepregnancy (mU/L)			Median (IQR)	Mean (SD)	Median (IQR)
Control	NA	NA	2.12 (1.50, 2.80)	0.652 (0.418)	2.00 (1.36, 2.70)
LT4	NA	NA	2.94 (2.04, 3.74)	0.674 (0.422)	2.10 (1.40, 3.11)
TSH trimester 1 (mU/L)	Mean (SD)	Mean (SD)	—	Mean (SD)	Median (IQR)
Control	1.7 (0.5)	1.37 (0.5)	NA	0.573 (0.766)	1.79 (1.30, 2.68)
LT4	1.6 (0.5)	1.42 (0.5)	NA	0.141 (0.967)*	1.37 (0.65, 2.16)**
TSH trimester 2 (mU/L)	Mean (SD)	Mean (SD)	—	Mean (SD)	Median (IQR)
Control	2.3 (0.5)	1.8 (0.8)	NA	0.385 (0.626)	1.90 (1.14, 2.40)
LT4	1.1 (0.4)*	1.23 (0.5)*	NA	0.177 (0.634)*	1.52 (0.92, 1.93)**
TSH trimester 3 (mU/L)	Mean (SD)	Mean (SD)	—	Mean (SD)	—
Control	2.5 (0.6)	2.49 (1.1)	NA	0.327 (0.519)	NA
LT4	1.2 (0.4)*	1.47 (0.8)*	NA	0.123 (0.552)*	NA

Primary trial outcome in **bold**. Difference between control and LT4 groups not statistically significant unless indicated by * (*P* < .05). For **, study text indicates value is lower than control but does not provide statistics.

Abbreviations: ART, assisted reproductive technologies; IQR, interquartile range; IVF, in vitro fertilization; LT4, levothyroxine; RPL, recurrent pregnancy loss; SD, standard deviation; TPOAb, thyroid peroxidase antibody; TSH, thyroid-stimulating hormone.

Power calculations.

Negro 2016: N = 318 needed to detect a 50% decrease in miscarriage (from 24% to 12%).

POSTAL: N = 600 needed to have 80% power to detect a 50% decrease in miscarriage rates (from 30% to 15%).

TABLET: N = 900 needed to have 80% power to detect 10% difference in live birth rates (from 55% to 65%).

T4LIFE: N = 240 needed to have 80% power to detect 20% difference in live birth rates (from 55% to 75%).

[a] Study did not define a primary outcome.

[b] 49% of "no treatment" group received treatment with LT4 starting in trimesters 2 or 3, when TSH >3.0 mU/L.

[c] 10% discontinued trial agent because of abnormal TFTs.

[d] 9% discontinued trial because of hypothyroidism.

[e] Trial stopped prematurely, not meeting recruitment goals.

miscarriage or subfertility randomized to 50 mcg LT4 preconception and throughout pregnancy had no difference in live births after 34 weeks.[50] Similar data were obtained in the POSTAL trial,[49] which randomized 600 subfertile women undergoing ART, and the T4LIFE trial,[51] investigating the effect of LT4 in 187 women with recurrent miscarriage history. All 3 RCTs had significant limitations, such as studying very specific yet varied populations of women, limited power to detect clinically relevant differences in important subgroups, and including women with borderline thyroid autoimmunity and TSH in the lower range of normal, which might have diluted the potential benefit of LT4 (see **Table 2**). In fact, median TSH was well below 2.5 mU/L at enrollment and stayed less than 2.5 mU/L in all trimesters in the studies that checked serial values, while the mean TSH was less than 0.7 mU/L at enrollment and stayed less than 0.6 mU/L throughout pregnancy in the placebo group in the TABLET study.[50] Thyroid antibody titers were assessed with 22 different assays in the TABLET trial and 15 assays in the T4LIFE trial and all borderline or indeterminate values were considered positive. This could have resulted in misclassification of patients without true thyroid autoimmunity in the study group, biasing results toward the null hypothesis. Nevertheless, the recent RCTs suggest that relative thyroid insufficiency is not the only mechanism at play in euthyroid women with thyroid autoimmunity, but there are likely multiple pathogenetic pathways involved, in different patient populations, and depending on the severity of the thyroid destruction.

The TABLET, POSTAL and T4LIFE RCTs, despite their limitations, all show that treatment of euthyroid TPOAb+ women with TSH less than 2.5 mU/L and history of infertility, miscarriage, RPL, or undergoing ART do not benefit from LT4 treatment. The results are consistent with prior ATA pregnancy guidelines that do not support treatment of this population and in fact do not recommend TPOAb testing for TSH less than 2.5 mU/L.[1] It is important to note, however, that these studies do not have sufficient data to address the effect of treatment in women with TSH 2.5 to 4.0 mU/L, or in certain subsets such as women with spontaneous pregnancy versus ART, women with very high TPOAb titers, or women with limited thyroid reserve. In fact, a recent meta-analysis showed that LT4 treatment reduced the risk of pregnancy loss (RR 0.61 [95% CI 0.39–0.96]) and preterm birth (RR 0.49 [95% CI 0.30–0.79]) in women with thyroid autoimmunity undergoing natural conception but not in pregnancies achieved through ART (RR 0.68 [95% CI 0.40–1.15] and RR 1.20 [95% CI 0.68–2.13], respectively).[52] Another meta-analysis raises the possibility that only women with high TPOAb titers might be at risk for miscarriage and therefore benefit from treatment. Miscarriage rates were not elevated in women when a TPOAb cutoff of greater than 34 IU/mL was used to define positivity (RR 0.61 [95% CI 0.35–1.08]) while they were significantly elevated when a cutoff of greater than 100 IU/mL was used (RR 2.12 [95% CI 1.52–2.96]).[53] There could also be a subgroup of women in whom thyroid autoimmunity causes a limited thyroid reserve, and who would thus benefit from LT4 treatment. In a study of patients with thyroid autoimmunity and preterm delivery, the FT4 response to HCG was found to be associated with the risk for preterm delivery. TPOAb+ women who had an expected FT4 response to HCG did not have increased rates of preterm delivery (OR 0.56), whereas those with suboptimal response to HCG had an OR greater than 2 for preterm delivery.[44] It is possible that LT4 treatment would benefit the latter group, but not the former. Finally, the follow-up to the TABLET trial has yielded some important information regarding the risk of developing hypothyroidism in women with thyroid autoimmunity in the short term and the implications of lack of treatment. When the TABLET participants were followed for 1 year after enrollment, 7.4% developed SCH or OH (27 out of 470 in the LT4 group vs 43 out of 470 in the placebo group): 84% preconception (most in the first 3 months) and 16% in the first trimester of pregnancy.[54] Baseline TSH and TPOAb levels were predictive of the development of SCH/OH (TSH 3 mU/L in patients who developed SCH/OH vs 2 mU/L in those who didn't, TPOAb 213 IU/mL vs 182 IU/mL), while LT4 treatment preconception reduced the occurrence of SCH/OH by 40%.[54] In subgroup analysis, the group of women with untreated SCH (N = 20) was found to have a lower chance of live birth compared with the group of women with treated SCH/OH (N = 50; RR 0.31 [95% CI 0.10–0.91]).[54] Given the earlier data suggesting that the population of euthyroid women with thyroid autoimmunity is not uniform, as well as the limitations of existing RCTs, further studies are needed to identify the subsets of euthyroid TPOAb$^+$ women that may benefit from LT4 treatment during pregnancy.

Treatment Recommendations/Considerations

The most recent clinical guidelines recommend treatment of all pregnant women with OH and pregnant women with SCH with TSH greater than 10 mU/L, with a goal TSH between the lower limit of the trimester-specific reference range and 2.5 mU/L.[1] For women with TSH less than 10 mU/L, the American Congress of Obstetricians and Gynecologists does not recommend treatment[55] and the ATA recommendations depend on the TPOAb status.[1] For women with TPOAb positivity, LT4 treatment is recommended for TSH between the upper limit of pregnancy-specific reference range (ULRR) and 10 mU/L and is to be considered for TSH between 2.5 mU/L and the ULRR. In women without thyroid autoimmunity, they recommend to consider treatment in those with TSH between the ULRR and 10 mU/L.[1] Our opinion is that LT4 treatment of all pregnant women with TSH greater than 4 mU/L is justified based on the evidence we presented in this review. For euthyroid women with thyroid autoimmunity further research is needed to identify whether there are certain subgroups that may benefit from LT4 therapy.

In addition to treatment algorithms, awareness of TPOAb positivity is critical in pregnancy. For TPOAb$^+$ women who are euthyroid prepregnancy, knowledge of the underlying autoimmunity allows for appropriate monitoring for the development of hypothyroidism preconception, during pregnancy, and in the postpartum phase. Monitoring thyroid function every 3 months preconception can promptly diagnose SCH/OH, if it occurs. During pregnancy, ATA guidelines recommend thyroid function monitoring every 4 weeks until midgestation, while therapy with LT4 should be initiated if SCH/OH develops.[1] These women should also be educated about the possibility of postpartum thyroiditis and have thyroid function assessed at regular intervals in the postpartum year.[1] Importantly, women with Hashimoto's disease who undergo ART can have significant alterations in thyroid tests in the process and before conception, as a result of the hormonal preparations needed in their fertility cycles.[56,57] Evaluation of thyroid function should be performed ideally before hormonal manipulation starts or a few weeks after controlled ovarian hyperstimulation, as the results at other times may be difficult to interpret.[1]

SUMMARY AND FUTURE DIRECTIONS

SCH is associated with adverse maternal and offspring outcomes. LT4 has been shown to improve pregnancy outcomes in women with TSH greater than 4 mU/L, but this effect was not found in RCTs with mean gestational age at randomization after the first trimester. Thyroid autoimmunity is associated with infertility and adverse obstetric outcomes independent of thyroid dysfunction. Existing studies, however, do not offer definitive answers for the potential benefit of treatment of euthyroid women with thyroid autoimmunity. Nevertheless, recent RCTs suggest that there is no clear obstetrical benefit to treating women with TSH less than 2.5 mU/L. To develop new evidence-based recommendations for patients with TSH 2.5 to 4.0 mU/L who are TPOAb[+], further studies are needed to determine:

a. what are the effects of LT4 on obstetrical outcomes in patients with thyroid auto-immunity and TSH 2.5 to 4.0 mU/L?
b. Are there different outcomes in patients with high TPOAb levels?
c. Are there different outcomes in spontaneous versus ART pregnancies?
d. What factors predict the development of SCH/OH during gestation in women with thyroid autoimmunity?
e. Are there ways to assess thyroidal reserve preconception?

A starting point could be to combine IPD from the TABLET, POSTAL, and T4LIFE trials for analysis, as recruitment for large RCTs in pregnancy is challenging. In addition, it would be useful to develop a way to test the adequacy of thyroid reserve in patients with thyroid autoimmunity in efforts to predict which patients would be able to mount an appropriate HCG response to fulfill the demands of pregnancy.

CLINICS CARE POINTS

- Women with SCH should be treated with LT4 if TSH is greater than 4.0 mU/L.
- Women with thyroid autoimmunity should be monitored with regular thyroid function tests preconception and during gestation.
- Further research is needed to identify whether there are subgroups of euthyroid women with thyroid autoimmunity who may benefit from LT4 therapy.

DISCLOSURE

The authors have nothing to disclose.

REFERENCES

1. Alexander EK, Pearce EN, Brent GA, et al. 2017 Guidelines of the American Thyroid Association for the Diagnosis and Management of Thyroid Disease During Pregnancy and the Postpartum. Thyroid 2017;27(3):315–89.
2. Dong AC, Stagnaro-Green A. Differences in Diagnostic Criteria Mask the True Prevalence of Thyroid Disease in Pregnancy: A Systematic Review and Meta-Analysis. Thyroid 2019;29(2):278–89.
3. Maraka S, Ospina NM, O'Keeffe DT, et al. Subclinical Hypothyroidism in Pregnancy: A Systematic Review and Meta-Analysis. Thyroid 2016;26(4):580–90.
4. Hollowell JG, Staehling NW, Flanders WD, et al. Serum TSH, T(4), and thyroid antibodies in the United States population (1988 to 1994): National Health and Nutrition Examination Survey (NHANES III). J Clin Endocrinol Metab 2002;87(2):489–99.
5. De Leo S, Pearce EN. Autoimmune thyroid disease during pregnancy. Lancet Diabetes Endocrinol 2018;6(7):575–86.
6. Glinoer D, Riahi M, Grun JP, et al. Risk of subclinical hypothyroidism in pregnant women with asymptomatic autoimmune thyroid disorders. J Clin Endocrinol Metab 1994;79(1):197–204.
7. Bliddal S, Derakhshan A, Xiao Y, et al. Association of Thyroid Peroxidase Antibodies and Thyroglobulin Antibodies with Thyroid Function in Pregnancy: An Individual Participant Data Meta-Analysis. Thyroid 2022;32(7):828–40.

8. Sun J, Teng D, Li C, et al. Association between iodine intake and thyroid autoantibodies: a cross-sectional study of 7073 early pregnant women in an iodine-adequate region. J Endocrinol Invest 2020;43(1):43–51.
9. Fowden AL, Forhead AJ. Endocrine mechanisms of intrauterine programming. Reproduction 2004;127(5):515–26.
10. Bernal J, Nunez J. Thyroid hormones and brain development. Eur J Endocrinol 1995;133(4):390–8.
11. Consortium on Thyroid and Pregnancy-Study Group on Preterm Birth, Korevaar T, Derakhshan A, Taylor PN, et al. Association of Thyroid Function Test Abnormalities and Thyroid Autoimmunity With Preterm Birth: A Systematic Review and Meta-analysis. JAMA 2019;322(7):632–41.
12. Toloza FJK, Derakhshan A, Mannisto T, et al. Association between maternal thyroid function and risk of gestational hypertension and pre-eclampsia: a systematic review and individual-participant data meta-analysis. Lancet Diabetes Endocrinol 2022;10(4):243–52.
13. Derakhshan A, Peeters RP, Taylor PN, et al. Association of maternal thyroid function with birthweight: a systematic review and individual-participant data meta-analysis. Lancet Diabetes Endocrinol 2020;8(6):501–10.
14. Thompson W, Russell G, Baragwanath G, et al. Maternal thyroid hormone insufficiency during pregnancy and risk of neurodevelopmental disorders in offspring: A systematic review and meta-analysis. Clin Endocrinol (Oxf) 2018;88(4):575–84.
15. Liu Y, Chen H, Jing C, et al. The Association Between Maternal Subclinical Hypothyroidism and Growth, Development, and Childhood Intelligence: A Meta-analysis. J Clin Res Pediatr Endocrinol 2018;10(2):153–61.
16. Levie D, Korevaar T, Mulder TA, et al. Maternal Thyroid Function in Early Pregnancy and Child Attention-Deficit Hyperactivity Disorder: An Individual-Participant Meta-Analysis. Thyroid 2019;29(9):1316–26.
17. Negro R, Schwartz A, Gismondi R, et al. Universal screening versus case finding for detection and treatment of thyroid hormonal dysfunction during pregnancy. J Clin Endocrinol Metab 2010;95(4):1699–707.
18. Lazarus JH, Bestwick JP, Channon S, et al. Antenatal thyroid screening and childhood cognitive function. N Engl J Med 2012;366(6):493–501.
19. Hales C, Taylor PN, Channon S, et al. Controlled Antenatal Thyroid Screening II: Effect of Treating Maternal Suboptimal Thyroid Function on Child Cognition. J Clin Endocrinol Metab 2018;103(4):1583–91.
20. Casey BM, Thom EA, Peaceman AM, et al. Treatment of Subclinical Hypothyroidism or Hypothyroxinemia in Pregnancy. N Engl J Med 2017;376(9):815–25.
21. Nazarpour S, Ramezani Tehrani F, Simbar M, et al. Effects of Levothyroxine on Pregnant Women With Subclinical Hypothyroidism, Negative for Thyroid Peroxidase Antibodies. J Clin Endocrinol Metab 2018;103(3):926–35.
22. Nazarpour S, Ramezani Tehrani F, Simbar M, et al. Effects of levothyroxine treatment on pregnancy outcomes in pregnant women with autoimmune thyroid disease. Eur J Endocrinol 2017;176(2):253–65.
23. Nazarpour S, Ramezani Tehrani F, Sajedi F, et al. Lack of beneficiary effect of levothyroxine therapy of pregnant women with subclinical hypothyroidism in terms of neurodevelopment of their offspring. Arch Gynecol Obstet 2024;309(3):975–85.
24. Maraka S, Mwangi R, McCoy RG, et al. Thyroid hormone treatment among pregnant women with subclinical hypothyroidism: US national assessment. BMJ 2017;356:i6865.
25. Burrow GN, Fisher DA, Larsen PR. Maternal and fetal thyroid function. N Engl J Med 1994;331(16):1072–8.

26. Mandel SJ, Larsen PR, Seely EW, et al. Increased need for thyroxine during pregnancy in women with primary hypothyroidism. N Engl J Med 1990;323(2):91–6.
27. Kaplan MM. Monitoring thyroxine treatment during pregnancy. Thyroid. Summer 1992;2(2):147–52.
28. Alexander EK, Marqusee E, Lawrence J, et al. Timing and magnitude of increases in levothyroxine requirements during pregnancy in women with hypothyroidism. N Engl J Med 2004;351(3):241–9.
29. Negro R, Formoso G, Mangieri T, et al. Levothyroxine treatment in euthyroid pregnant women with autoimmune thyroid disease: effects on obstetrical complications. J Clin Endocrinol Metab 2006;91(7):2587–91.
30. Leber A, Teles A, Zenclussen AC. Regulatory T cells and their role in pregnancy. Am J Reprod Immunol 2010;63(6):445–59.
31. Feldt-Rasmussen U, Hoier-Madsen M, Rasmussen NG, et al. Anti-thyroid peroxidase antibodies during pregnancy and postpartum. Relation to postpartum thyroiditis. Autoimmunity 1990;6(3):211–4.
32. Premawardhana LD, Parkes AB, Ammari F, et al. Postpartum thyroiditis and long-term thyroid status: prognostic influence of thyroid peroxidase antibodies and ultrasound echogenicity. J Clin Endocrinol Metab 2000;85(1):71–5.
33. Premawardhana LD, Parkes AB, John R, et al. Thyroid peroxidase antibodies in early pregnancy: utility for prediction of postpartum thyroid dysfunction and implications for screening. Thyroid 2004;14(8):610–5.
34. Quintino-Moro A, Zantut-Wittmann DE, Tambascia M, et al. High Prevalence of Infertility among Women with Graves' Disease and Hashimoto's Thyroiditis. Int J Endocrinol 2014;2014:982705.
35. Chen CW, Huang YL, Tzeng CR, et al. Idiopathic Low Ovarian Reserve Is Associated with More Frequent Positive Thyroid Peroxidase Antibodies. Thyroid 2017; 27(9):1194–200.
36. Korevaar T, Minguez-Alarcon L, Messerlian C, et al. Association of Thyroid Function and Autoimmunity with Ovarian Reserve in Women Seeking Infertility Care. Thyroid 2018;28(10):1349–58.
37. Seungdamrong A, Steiner AZ, Gracia CR, et al. Preconceptional antithyroid peroxidase antibodies, but not thyroid-stimulating hormone, are associated with decreased live birth rates in infertile women. Fertil Steril 2017;S0015-0282(17): 31748-X.
38. Stagnaro-Green A, Roman SH, Cobin RH, et al. Detection of at-risk pregnancy by means of highly sensitive assays for thyroid autoantibodies. JAMA 1990;264(11): 1422–5.
39. Thangaratinam S, Tan A, Knox E, et al. Association between thyroid autoantibodies and miscarriage and preterm birth: meta-analysis of evidence. BMJ 2011;342:d2616.
40. Chen L, Hu R. Thyroid autoimmunity and miscarriage: a meta-analysis. Clin Endocrinol (Oxf) 2011;74(4):513–9.
41. Liu H, Shan Z, Li C, et al. Maternal subclinical hypothyroidism, thyroid autoimmunity, and the risk of miscarriage: a prospective cohort study. Thyroid 2014;24(11): 1642–9.
42. Xie J, Jiang L, Sadhukhan A, et al. Effect of antithyroid antibodies on women with recurrent miscarriage: A meta-analysis. Am J Reprod Immunol 2020;83(6):e13238.
43. Abbassi-Ghanavati M, Casey BM, Spong CY, et al. Pregnancy outcomes in women with thyroid peroxidase antibodies. Obstet Gynecol 2010;116(2 Pt 1): 381–6.

44. Korevaar T, Steegers EA, Pop VJ, et al. Thyroid Autoimmunity Impairs the Thyroidal Response to Human Chorionic Gonadotropin: Two Population-Based Prospective Cohort Studies. J Clin Endocrinol Metab 2017;102(1):69–77.
45. Monteleone P, Faviana P, Artini PG. Thyroid peroxidase identified in human granulosa cells: another piece to the thyroid-ovary puzzle? Gynecol Endocrinol 2017; 33(7):574–6.
46. Miko E, Meggyes M, Doba K, et al. Characteristics of peripheral blood NK and NKT-like cells in euthyroid and subclinical hypothyroid women with thyroid autoimmunity experiencing reproductive failure. J Reprod Immunol 2017;124:62–70.
47. Andrisani A, Sabbadin C, Marin L, et al. The influence of thyroid autoimmunity on embryo quality in women undergoing assisted reproductive technology. Gynecol Endocrinol 2018;34(9):752–5.
48. Negro R, Schwartz A, Stagnaro-Green A. Impact of Levothyroxine in Miscarriage and Preterm Delivery Rates in First Trimester Thyroid Antibody-Positive Women With TSH Less Than 2.5 mIU/L. J Clin Endocrinol Metab 2016;101(10):3685–90.
49. Wang H, Gao H, Chi H, et al. Effect of Levothyroxine on Miscarriage Among Women With Normal Thyroid Function and Thyroid Autoimmunity Undergoing In Vitro Fertilization and Embryo Transfer: A Randomized Clinical Trial. JAMA 2017;318(22):2190–8.
50. Dhillon-Smith RK, Middleton LJ, Sunner KK, et al. Levothyroxine in Women with Thyroid Peroxidase Antibodies before Conception. N Engl J Med 2019;380(14): 1316–25.
51. van Dijk MM, Vissenberg R, Fliers E, et al. Levothyroxine in euthyroid thyroid peroxidase antibody positive women with recurrent pregnancy loss (T4LIFE trial): a multicentre, randomised, double-blind, placebo-controlled, phase 3 trial. Lancet Diabetes Endocrinol 2022;10(5):322–9.
52. Rao M, Zeng Z, Zhou F, et al. Effect of levothyroxine supplementation on pregnancy loss and preterm birth in women with subclinical hypothyroidism and thyroid autoimmunity: a systematic review and meta-analysis. Hum Reprod Update 2019;25(3):344–61.
53. Zhang S, Yang M, Li T, et al. High level of thyroid peroxidase antibodies as a detrimental risk of pregnancy outcomes in euthyroid women undergoing ART: A meta-analysis. Mol Reprod Dev 2023;90(4):218–26.
54. Gill S, Cheed V, Morton VAH, et al. Evaluating the Progression to Hypothyroidism in Preconception Euthyroid Thyroid Peroxidase Antibody-Positive Women. J Clin Endocrinol Metab 2022;108(1):124–34.
55. American College of O, Gynecologists' Committee on Practice B-O. Thyroid Disease in Pregnancy: ACOG Practice Bulletin, Number 223. Obstet Gynecol 2020; 135(6):e261–74.
56. Li L, Li L, Li P. Effects of controlled ovarian stimulation on thyroid function during pregnancydagger. Biol Reprod 2022;107(6):1376–85.
57. Busnelli A, Cirillo F, Levi-Setti PE. Thyroid function modifications in women undergoing controlled ovarian hyperstimulation for in vitro fertilization: a systematic review and meta-analysis. Fertil Steril 2021;116(1):218–31.

Update on Preeclampsia and Hypertensive Disorders of Pregnancy

Emily A. Rosenberg, MD[a], Ellen W. Seely, MD[b],*

KEYWORDS

- Women's health • Preeclampsia • Hypertensive disorders of pregnancy • Aspirin
- Cardiovascular disease

KEY POINTS

- Preeclampsia, a hypertensive disorder of pregnancy, is a multisystem disease and remains a leading cause of maternal and fetal/neonatal morbidity and mortality in the United States.
- The use of low-dose aspirin, optimally initiated before 16 weeks' gestation, reduces the risk of preterm (<37 weeks gestation) preeclampsia in high-risk women.
- The use of the soluble fms-like tyrosine kinase 1/placental growth factor ratio has been Food and Drug Administration approved for the short-term prediction of preeclampsia.
- The outcomes of pregnancies complicated by chronic hypertension are improved if antihypertensives are initiated at a threshold of 140/90 mm Hg rather than the previous endorsed threshold of 160/110 mm Hg.
- Women with a history of preeclampsia and gestational hypertension have increased risk for future cardiovascular disease and therefore should receive risk reduction counseling.

INTRODUCTION

Hypertensive disorders of pregnancy (HDPs) complicate approximately 16% of pregnancies in the United States (U.S.).[1] HDPs, according to the American College of Obstetrics and Gynecology (ACOG),[2,3] include new-onset hypertension in pregnancy, typically in the second half of pregnancy, in the form of preeclampsia (hypertension with end organ damage) or gestational hypertension (hypertension alone), preeclampsia superimposed on chronic pre-pregnancy hypertension, and chronic hypertension (**Table 1**).

---

[a] Division of Endocrinology, Diabetes, and Metabolic Diseases, Medical University of South Carolina, 96 Jonathan Lucas Street, CSB 822, Charleston, SC 29425, USA; [b] Department of Medicine, Division of Endocrinology, Diabetes, and Hypertension, Brigham & Women's Hospital, Harvard Medical School, 221 Longwood Avenue, Boston, MA 02115, USA
* Corresponding author.
E-mail address: eseely@bwh.harvard.edu

Endocrinol Metab Clin N Am 53 (2024) 377–389
https://doi.org/10.1016/j.ecl.2024.05.012
0889-8529/24/© 2024 Elsevier Inc. All rights reserved, including those for text and data mining, AI training, and similar technologies.
endo.theclinics.com

Table 1
Hypertensive disorders of pregnancy definitions adapted from the American College of Obstetricians and Gynecologists (Practice Bulletins 203 and 222[2,3])

	Definition

Preeclampsia	• New-onset hypertension
	  ○ Systolic blood pressure of $\geq$ 140 mm Hg and/or diastolic blood pressure $\geq$ 90 mm Hg on 2 occasions at least 4 hours apart after 20 weeks of gestation in a woman with a previously normal blood pressure.
	• And new-onset (any 1 of the following):
	  ○ Proteinuria: $\geq$ 300 mg/24-hour urine (or this amount extrapolated from a timed collection) or protein/creatinine ratio of $\geq$ 0.3 or dipstick reading of $\geq$ 2+ (used only if other quantitative methods not available)
	  ○ Thrombocytopenia: Platelet count<100 x 10^9/L
	  ○ Renal insufficiency: Serum creatinine concentrations>1.1 mg/dL or a doubling of serum creatinine concentration in absence of other renal disease
	  ○ Impaired liver function: Elevated concentrations of liver transaminases 2 times normal concentration
	  ○ Pulmonary edema
	  ○ New-onset headache not responsive to medication and not accounted for by alternative diagnoses or visual symptoms

Preeclampsia with severe features	• Presence of any of the following findings are features of severe disease:
	  ○ Systolic blood pressure $\geq$ 160 and/or diastolic blood pressure $\geq$ 110 on 2 occasions at least 4 hours apart (unless individual is already on antihypertensive therapy)
	  ○ Thrombocytopenia: Platelet count<100 x 10^9/L
	  ○ Renal insufficiency: Serum creatinine concentrations>1.1 mg/dL or a doubling of serum creatinine concentration in absence of other renal disease
	  ○ Impaired liver function (elevated concentrations of liver transaminases 2 times normal concentration or severe persistent right upper quadrant or epigastric pain not responsive to medications)
	  ○ Pulmonary edema
	  ○ New-onset headache not responsive to medication and not accounted for by alternative diagnoses
	  ○ Visual disturbances

Gestational hypertension	• New-onset hypertension
	  ○ Systolic blood pressure $\geq$140 mm Hg and/or diastolic blood pressure $\geq$ 90 mm Hg on 2 occasions at least 4 hours apart after 20 weeks of gestation in a woman with a previously normal blood pressure[a]
	  ○ Without proteinuria or signs/symptoms of preeclampsia-related end-organ dysfunction

Chronic hypertension	• Hypertension[b] diagnosed or present before pregnancy or before 20 weeks of gestation Or • Hypertension that is diagnosed for the first time during pregnancy and that does not resolve in the postpartum period.
Preeclampsia superimposed on chronic pre-pregnancy hypertension	• Preeclampsia is considered superimposed when it complicates preexisting chronic hypertension.

[a] Women with gestational hypertension with blood pressure in the severe range should be diagnosed with preeclampsia with severe features.
[b] Blood pressure criteria during pregnancy are systolic blood pressure $\geq$140 mm Hg and/or diastolic blood pressure $\geq$90 mm Hg. Pre-pregnancy and postpartum blood pressure criteria are systolic blood pressure $\geq$130 mm Hg and/or diastolic blood pressure $\geq$80 mm Hg.[2,3]

HDPs account for 16.9% of all pregnancy-related maternal deaths in the United States.[4] The incidence of preeclampsia is 2% to 8%.[3] Preeclampsia is a multisystem disease and is associated with the development of myocardial infarction, stroke, acute respiratory distress syndrome, pulmonary edema, renal failure, coagulopathy, and seizures (termed eclampsia) in the mother.[3,5] Risks for the fetus include fetal growth restriction with resultant small for gestational age and iatrogenic prematurity, as the only cure for preeclampsia is delivery, which may need to occur regardless of gestational age, in order to save the life of the mother. Risks for developing preeclampsia include prior preeclampsia, chronic hypertension, pregestational diabetes, renal disease, autoimmune disease, and multiple pregnancies.[6] Preeclampsia resolves with delivery; however, women who have experienced preeclampsia have increased risk of future hypertension, heart disease, stroke, and cardiovascular mortality.[7]

Although the etiology of preeclampsia remains poorly understood and curative treatments other than delivery remain unavailable, advances have been made in the past decade in the care of women with preeclampsia and HDPs. Some of these advances include (1) the use of low-dose aspirin (acetylsalicylic acid [ASA]) for the prevention of preeclampsia, (2) the use of soluble fms-like tyrosine kinase 1 (sFlt-1)/placental growth factor (PIGF) ratio for the short-term prediction of preeclampsia, (3) the revision of blood pressure (BP) goals for initiating antihypertensives in pregnancy, and (4) the incorporation of preeclampsia and gestational hypertension as cardiovascular risk factors in women.

PREVENTION OF PREECLAMPSIA

For decades, there has been a search to identify interventions that could decrease preeclampsia risk, especially preterm preeclampsia. In 2017, researchers revisited the use of low-dose ASA for the prevention of preterm preeclampsia (development of preeclampsia before 37 weeks' gestation) in high-risk women. The Aspirin for Evidence-Based Preeclampsia Prevention randomized controlled multicenter trial of ASA versus placebo was conducted in 1620 high-risk women.[8] The participants were defined as high risk based on an algorithm combining maternal risk factors, mean arterial pressure, uterine pulsatility index, and maternal levels of serum pregnancy-associated plasma protein and PIGF. The study population was over 65% white, approximately 25% black, and 6% Asian. The intervention group received 150 mg of ASA at bedtime from 11 to 14 weeks of gestation to 36 weeks of gestation. The arm which received ASA had a rate of preterm preeclampsia of 1.6% whereas the placebo arm had a rate of 4.3% ($P = .004$ between groups) (**Fig. 1**). There was no decrease in the risk of term preeclampsia. Adverse events were similar between groups and analysis by subgroup indicated benefit to all subgroups except in women with chronic hypertension.

Regarding potential adverse effects associated with ASA use in pregnancy, recent studies have not shown an increased risk of postpartum hemorrhage.[8,9] However, an increase in the risk of cerebral palsy was found in a study from Denmark,[10] but not in other studies. Drawbacks to the Danish study include lack of adjustment for preterm birth, a leading cause of cerebral palsy. Promisingly, a questionnaire study concerning offsprings of mothers exposed to ASA showed no adverse effects on offsprings up to 18 months of age.[11]

The mechanism by which ASA decreases preeclampsia risk is not yet established. There are several putative mechanisms. Low-dose ASA inhibits cyclooxygenase 1 (COX-1) resulting in decreased platelet synthesis of thromboxane A2 without inhibition of COX-2 so maintenance of prostacyclin synthesis by the vessel wall results in a more antithrombotic milieu.[12] Low-dose ASA may also modify cytokine secretion leading to

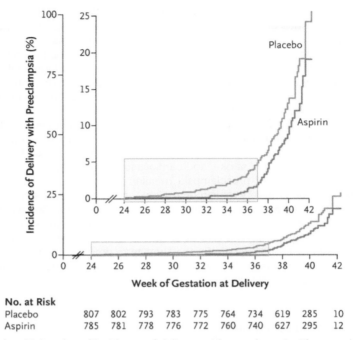

No. at Risk

Placebo		807	802	793	783	775	764	734	619	285	10
Aspirin		785	781	778	776	772	760	740	627	295	12

Fig. 1. Kaplan–Meier plot of incidence of delivery with preeclampsia: The cumulative percentages of participants who had delivery with preeclampsia in the low-dose aspirin (acetylsalicylic acid [ASA]) arm (*red*) versus the placebo arm (*blue*). The gray box highlights the rate of preeclampsia before 37 weeks of gestation. Data were censored after deliveries not associated with preeclampsia. The inset shows the same data on an enlarged y-axis. (*From* The New England Journal of Medicine, Rolnik DL et al., Aspirin versus Placebo in Pregnancies at High Risk for Preterm Preeclampsia. 2017 Aug 17;377(7):613-622. Copyright © 2017 Massachusetts Medical Society. Reprinted with permission from Massachusetts Medical Society.)

reduced placental cell apoptosis.[13] There are other effects induced by low-dose ASA that may decrease inflammation and improve placentation and endothelial function.[14]

Because of these clinical trial findings, many societies have incorporated the use of ASA into prevention of preterm preeclampsia guidelines. There are many similarities to these guidelines/recommendations, but they differ in terms of the dose of ASA specified, the weeks of gestation that ASA should be initiated, whether the time of day for dosing is indicated, whether or when the ASA should be stopped, and which women should receive low-dose ASA.

Although many societies recommend low-dose ASA for high-risk women, there are multiple challenges to the implementation of this evidence-based recommendation. In terms of dosing, 150 mg of ASA as a single dose is not available in some countries such as the United States and Canada. Several guidelines have adapted their recommendations by specifying a range in dose. A survey study in the United States found that only 58% of patients with risk factors recalled ever receiving a recommendation to take low-dose ASA.[15] To overcome these barriers, the Society for Maternal-Fetal Medicine has published a quality metric to increase the rate of appropriate prescribing of ASA.[16] Some suggestions include educational materials for providers reminding them of eligibility criteria, the use of a provider check list,[17] electronic medical record–based reminders to providers,[18] and systematic feedback to providers on prescribing patterns.

ANGIOGENIC FACTORS TO PREDICT THE RISK OF PREECLAMPSIA

An imbalance of soluble sFlt-1 and PlGF has been reported in women after diagnosis with preeclampsia as well as prior to the development of preeclampsia.[19] Based on this observation, the hope was that these levels individually or as a ratio would be able to predict which women would develop preeclampsia. Studies using these levels alone or as a ratio in early pregnancy to predict preeclampsia have not supported their predictive value. However, in 2016, Zeisler and colleagues[20] studied the value of the ratio in later pregnancy to rule out the development of preeclampsia in women with suspected preeclampsia. The study demonstrated that a sFlt-1/PlGF ratio ≤38 was accurate in ruling out the development of preeclampsia in the next 2 weeks with a high negative predictive value (NPV) of 99.3% [97.9–99.9] (sensitivity 80% and specificity 78.3%). The positive predictive value (PPV) was only 36.7% [28.4–45.7] (sensitivity 66.2% and specificity 83.1%). This study suggested that a ratio lower than 38 could potentially reduce unnecessary hospitalization.

The subsequent randomized study, Interventional Study Evaluating the Short-Term Prediction of Preeclampsia/Eclampsia In Pregnant Women With Suspected Preeclampsia (INSPIRE), evaluated the use of sFlt-1/PlGF with a threshold of 38 to predict preeclampsia in 370 women with suspected preeclampsia.[21] In the intervention group, clinical providers were provided with the result of the ratio to use with clinical judgment; in the control group, the ratio was determined but not revealed so only clinical judgment could be used. The primary endpoint was hospitalization within 24 hours of the test and a secondary endpoint was the development of preeclampsia. There was no difference in the hospitalization rate. However, in the intervention arm, 100% of the women who developed preeclampsia within 7 days were admitted as compared to 83% in the control arm (P = .038). The NPV of the ratio ≤38 in combination with clinical judgment was 100% [97.1–100] (100% sensitivity) compared to tNPV of 97.8% [93.7–99.5] (83.3% sensitivity) with clinical judgment alone.

The US Food and Drug Administration approval for the ratio occurred in May 2023 based on results of the Preeclampsia Risk Assessment: Evaluation of Cut-offs to Improve Stratification (PRAECIS) multicenter blinded prospective study.[22] The PRAECIS study included over 700 pregnant women hospitalized for HDPs from 18 hospitals across the United States. In the validation cohort, a ratio of ≥40 was used to predict the development of preeclampsia in the next week as the primary outcome. The validation cohort population was diverse (30% black, 16% Hispanic). An sFlt-1/PlGF ratio of ≥40 demonstrated a 65% PPV (95% confidence interval [CI], 59–71) and a 96% NPV (95% CI, 93–98) for preeclampsia development in the next 2 weeks (**Fig. 2**). The strong NPV of the ratio may be helpful in ruling out preeclampsia with the potential to decrease the need for hospitalization and shorten hospitalizations for women with low ratios, resulting in cost savings.[23,24] Some societies have incorporated a recommendation for the use of this ratio in combination with standard clinical assessment into practice recommendations such as the Canadian National Institute for Health and Care Excellence.[25]

ANTIHYPERTENSIVE TREATMENT OF HYPERTENSION IN PREGNANCY: WHEN TO INITIATE THERAPY?

Treatment of hypertension during pregnancy requires considering the risks and benefits of treatment to both the pregnant individual and the fetus. There has been controversy regarding treatment goals and when to initiate therapy among individuals

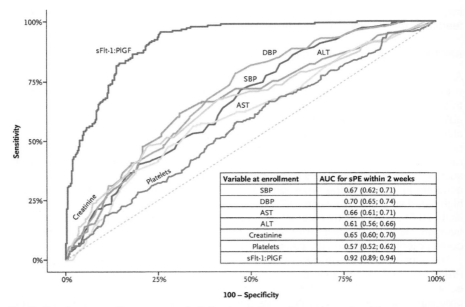

Variable at enrollment	AUC for sPE within 2 weeks
SBP	0.67 (0.62; 0.71)
DBP	0.70 (0.65; 0.74)
AST	0.66 (0.61; 0.71)
ALT	0.61 (0.56; 0.66)
Creatinine	0.65 (0.60; 0.70)
Platelets	0.57 (0.52; 0.62)
sFlt-1:PlGF	0.92 (0.89; 0.94)

Fig. 2. Receiver-operating curve analysis for prediction of preeclampsia with severe features (sPE) within 2 weeks using enrollment soluble fms-like tyrosine kinase 1 (sFlt-1):placental growth factor (PlGF) ratio, systolic and diastolic blood pressure (SBP and DBP, respectively), serum creatinine, aspartate aminotransferase (AST), alanine aminotransferase (ALT), and platelet counts. Panel (*inset*) depicts the area under the curve (AUC) for sFlt-1:PlGF ratio and all the standard-of-care clinical and biochemical tests. (*From* NEJM Evidence, Ravi Thadhani, M.D., M.P.H et al., Circulating Angiogenic Factor Levels in Hypertensive Disorders of Pregnancy, 1(12), 1-13. Copyright © 2022. Massachusetts Medical Society. Reprinted with permission from Massachusetts Medical Society.)

with hypertension due to concern for reduction in uteroplacental perfusion, fetal exposure to antihypertensive medication, and unclear benefit of tight BP control.[26,27]

While the definition of hypertension in pregnancy is uniform across guidelines (systolic BP of ≥140 mm Hg and/or diastolic BP of ≥90 mm Hg), guidelines vary in initiation of therapy thresholds with some guidelines recommending antihypertensive treatment in individuals with systolic BP ≥140 mm Hg and/or diastolic BP ≥90 mm Hg, while others do not initiate therapy until BP is in the severe range (≥160 mm Hg and/or diastolic BP ≥110 mm Hg).[27,28] While there is less agreement regarding the use of antihypertensives in individuals with BP<160/110 mm Hg, there is consensus for the treatment of individuals with severe hypertension. The ACOG currently recommends that any pregnant individual with severe hypertension (≥160 mm Hg and/or diastolic BP ≥110 mm Hg) confirmed by a repeat measurement (within 15 minutes) be initiated on antihypertensive therapy.[3]

Treatment of hypertension in pregnancy has used diagnostic thresholds above those in nonpregnant adults because of unclear benefit and concern for risk. Previous research has suggested an increased risk for small-for-gestational-age infants with the treatment of hypertension in the mild to moderate range.[29] A Cochrane review that compared treatment with antihypertensives to no treatment in over 3000 individuals with mild to moderate hypertension during pregnancy demonstrated a reduction in the development of severe hypertension but did not show a difference in the rates of preeclampsia, neonatal death, small for gestational age, or preterm birth.[30] Similarly, in the Control of Hypertension in Pregnancy Study (CHIPS) trial, where individuals with gestational hypertension or chronic hypertension were randomized to less-tight control (N = 493, target diastolic BP 100 mm Hg) or tight control (N = 488, target diastolic BP 85 mm Hg), severe hypertension developed in 40.6% of the individuals in the less-tight control group as compared to 27.5% of the individuals in the tight control group (P<.001).[31] However, there was no difference in the primary outcome between both groups, which was a composite of pregnancy loss or high-level neonatal care, and there was no difference in the rate of preeclampsia. More individuals in the less-tight control group experienced thrombocytopenia and elevated liver function tests, but these differences were not significant.

Reserving antihypertensive therapy for only women with BP in the severe range (≥160 mm Hg and/or diastolic BP ≥110 mm Hg) has been challenged by more recent data which show that the initiation of treatment at the lower threshold of 140/90 mm Hg in individuals with mild chronic hypertension is beneficial. In the Chronic Hypertension and Pregnancy (CHAP) Trial Consortium's randomized control trial, 2408 individuals with a new diagnosis of chronic hypertension (defined as a systolic BP of ≥140 mm Hg or diastolic BP of ≥90 mm Hg, or both on at least 2 occasions at least 4 hours apart before 20 weeks' gestation in patients without chronic hypertension) or known chronic hypertension (documentation of elevation in BP and previous or current antihypertensive therapy, including lifestyle measures) during pregnancy were randomized to the active treatment arm, where antihypertensives were initiated and the BP goal was less than 140/90 mm Hg, or to the standard treatment (control), in which antihypertensive therapy was withheld or stopped at randomization unless severe hypertension developed (≥160 mm Hg and/or diastolic BP ≥105 mm Hg). Of the 2408 individuals in the study, approximately 48% were non-Hispanic black, 20% were Hispanic, and 28% were non-Hispanic white. Results demonstrated that the incidence of the composite primary outcome, which included preeclampsia with severe features, medically indicated preterm birth before 35 weeks' gestation, placental abruption, or fetal or neonatal death was significantly lower in the active-treatment group than in the control group (30.2% vs 37%, adjusted risk ratio 0.82 (95% CI 0.74–0.92), P<.001) without a difference in the rates of small for gestational age.[32] The mean BP was lower in the active-treatment group than in the control group (systolic BP 129.5 mm Hg vs 132.6 mm Hg, and diastolic pressure 79.1 mm Hg vs 81.5 mm Hg). In subgroup analyses, individuals with diabetes (16% of the participants) showed a greater benefit from the lower treatment threshold (risk ratio 0.75, CI [0.59–0.94]) when compared to individuals without diabetes (risk ratio 0.84, CI [0.73–0.95]).[32] In further support of lower thresholds, a retrospective cohort study performed in China showed that individuals with chronic hypertension during pregnancy with lower BP (defined as diastolic BP<90) had lower incidences of small for gestational age, neonatal intensive care unit admission, preeclampsia with severe features, and severe hypertension than those with higher BP (defined as diastolic BP ≥ 90 mm Hg).[33] Individuals in the higher BP group delivered earlier and their infants had lower birth weight.[33] In a secondary analysis of the Community-Level Interventions for Preeclampsia trial, which included all types of HDPs, pregnant individuals from under-resourced settings were studied and classified using the 2017 American Heart Association (AHA) BP definitions.[34] The goal of this study was to explore a dose-response relationship between a wide range of BP categories and adverse outcomes. The investigators found that there was a dose-response relationship with the higher BP categories having a greater relative risk for adverse outcomes compared with normal BP. However, there was no increase in relative risk for adverse maternal, fetal, or neonatal outcomes seen in women with stage 1 hypertension (systolic BP 130–139 mm Hg and/

or diastolic BP 80–89) compared with women with normal BP. The increase in relative risk of adverse events began with stage 2 hypertension (systolic BP>140 and/or diastolic BP>90 mm Hg).[35]

Shortly after the publication of the CHAP trial in 2022, the ACOG released a statement recommending a BP of 140/90 mm Hg be used as the threshold for initiation of antihypertensive therapy among pregnant individuals with chronic hypertension rather than 160/110 mm Hg.[36] Similarly in 2022, the Society for Maternal-Fetal Medicine and the International Society for the Study of Hypertension in Pregnancy also released statements recommending treatment with antihypertensive therapy for mild chronic hypertension in pregnancy with a goal BP ofless than 140/90 mm Hg.[37,38] Prior to the publication of the CHAP trial, the AHA released a statement favoring a lower diagnostic and treatment threshold for HDPs more in line with stage 1 hypertension in nonpregnant adults (systolic BP $\geq$130 mm Hg or diastolic BP $\geq$80 mm Hg) but also recommended taking an individualized approach to the treatment of each patient given limited data.[28] Despite the findings from the CHAP study, more research is needed to determine how the findings from this trial may be applied to individuals with other forms of HDPs and whether initiating antihypertensives at a lower threshold in individuals with gestational hypertension or preeclampsia has similar clinical benefits.

LONG-TERM CONSEQUENCES FROM HYPERTENSIVE DISORDERS OF PREGNANCY

While HDPs were once thought of as conditions isolated to pregnancy, it is now known that these conditions impart an increased risk of future cardiovascular disease (CVD).[7] HDPs increase the risk of atherosclerotic CVD, including coronary heart disease, peripheral vascular disease, and ischemic stroke, as well as hemorrhagic stroke and heart failure.[7] In a recent meta-analysis that evaluated 83 studies, both gestational hypertension and preeclampsia were associated with cardiovascular-related morbidity, defined as coronary artery disease, myocardial infarction, coronary revascularization, peripheral arterial disease, transient ischemic attack, or stroke.[39] Pooled results of 9 studies demonstrated a 67% increased risk of the development of CVD in individuals with gestational hypertension when compared to women without gestational hypertension (CI [1.28–2.19]). Moderate preeclampsia (odds ratio 2.24, CI [1.72–2.93]) and severe preeclampsia (odds ratio 2.74 CI [2.48–3.04]) were associated with a significantly higher risk of cardiovascular-related morbidity as well.[39] Individuals with preeclampsia were also at higher risk of developing ischemic heart disease (odds ratio 1.73, CI [1.46–2.06]) and cerebrovascular disease (odds ratio 2.95, CI [1.10–7.90]). Moreover, preeclampsia was associated with a 75% increased risk of cardiovascular-related mortality (CI [1.46–2.06]). In another recent meta-analysis including 73 studies evaluating the relationship between history of HDPs and future risk of CVD, the pooled risk ratio was 1.80 (CI [1.67–1.94]).[40] There was a significantly increased risk of coronary heart disease (risk ratio 1.66, CI [1.49–1.84]), heart failure (risk ratio 2.87, CI [2.14–3.85]), peripheral vascular disease (risk ratio 1.60, CI [1.29–2.00]), and stroke (risk ratio 1.72, CI [1.50–1.97) among individuals with a history of HDPs compared to those without a history of HDPs. In a subgroup analysis, the risk of developing any form of CVD was higher among individuals with a history of preeclampsia (risk ratio 2.07, CI [1.86–2.30]) than in individuals with a history of gestational hypertension (risk ratio 1.64, CI [1.43–1.89]). The pooled risk estimate of CVD-related mortality among individuals with a history of HDP was 1.78 (CI [1.58–2.00]).[40]

It remains to be determined whether the relationship between preeclampsia and future CVD exists because preeclampsia unmasks traditional cardiovascular risk factors or whether it causes vascular damage that itself leads to CVD. In an analysis of the Nurse's Health Study, women who reported preeclampsia had a 63% higher rate of CVD (CI: 1.37–1.94) versus those with normotensive pregnancies even after adjustment for baseline CVD risk factors. Of note is the finding that traditional CVD risk factors (chronic hypertension, hypercholesterolemia, type 2 diabetes, and overweight/obesity) that developed after pregnancy accounted for 57% of the CVD risk in women with prior preeclampsia.[41] This finding suggests that traditional CVD risk factor reduction may decrease the risk for CVD. On the other hand, animal studies, which use experimental models of preeclampsia, have shown that pregnant mice randomized to receive sFlt-1 (which induces a phenotype of preeclampsia), as opposed to control pregnant mice, manifest salt sensitive BP and increased systemic BP and mesenteric vessel vasoconstriction in response to angiotensin II when studied 2 months after delivery.[42] These findings suggest that preeclampsia may induce long-lasting vascular changes associated with future CVD. More research is warranted to understand the mechanisms by which preeclampsia may induce risk for CVD and to develop approaches that could lessen this risk.

In 2011, the AHA released the "Effectiveness-Based Guidelines for the Prevention of Cardiovascular Disease in Women—2011 Update: A Guideline from the American Heart Association" and for the first time included preeclampsia as a major risk factor for CVD.[43] This guideline suggests that all parous women be asked about pregnancy complications such as preeclampsia so that risk factors for CVD can be both monitored and controlled. Recommendations to reduce the risk of CVD focus on lifestyle intervention for healthy eating, physical activity, weight reduction or maintenance, and smoking cessation.[43]

Given that at least some of the risk for CVD appears mediated by traditional risk factors, it is expected that risk factor reduction would reduce risk of CVD in this population. However, some women with prior preeclampsia are not aware of having had this diagnosis or of its link to future CVD[44] and clinical providers are often still not aware of this link[45,46] and do not provide cardiovascular risk reduction counseling as recommended by the AHA.[43] It is important that women who have had preeclampsia are made aware of their diagnosis so that they can let their future providers know. In a recent study, 88.3% of women who reported that a clinical provider had told them they had preeclampsia had their diagnosis validated with a clinician-documented diagnosis of preeclampsia in the medical record.[47]

Given the clear link between HDPs and other adverse pregnancy outcomes (APOs), the AHA issued a scientific statement in 2021 summarizing the evidence supporting this link.[7] The most recent AHA cholesterol treatment guidelines in 2018 now consider preeclampsia and other APOs that increase risk of CVD as risk-enhancing factors, which should be considered when deciding on whether or not to prescribe a statin for CVD prevention.[48] These findings underscore the importance of gathering a pregnancy history when assessing future CVD risk.

SUMMARY

HDPs are common conditions affecting pregnant women and are one of the major causes of maternal mortality in the United States. Recent research in the field has supported the use of aspirin as a preventative therapy for preeclampsia in high-risk women and has also elucidated new diagnostic tests for detecting preeclampsia, namely the sFlt-1/PlGF ratio. Recent research supports the use of antihypertensive therapy during pregnancy to target BP less than 140/90 mm Hg in women with chronic hypertension, challenging the traditional threshold of 160/110 mm Hg, but whether or not individuals with gestational hypertension or preeclampsia benefit from tighter BP control is unclear. It is now widely recognized that HDPs along with other APOs are risk factors for the future development of CVD and a history of these complications should be elicited in all women to help target risk reduction.

CLINICS CARE POINTS

- Low-dose aspirin should be prescribed to pregnant individuals at high risk for preeclampsia who do not have a contraindication before 16 weeks' gestation to reduce the risk of preterm preeclampsia. This includes both individuals with type 1 and type 2 diabetes.

- The soluble sFlt-1/PlGF ratio is a diagnostic tool to predict the short-term (over the next 2 weeks) development of preeclampsia in women with suspected preeclampsia. The ratio performs best in predicting those women who will not develop preeclampsia. The use of the ratio may shorten hospital stays.

- The CHAP trial demonstrated that initiating antihypertensive therapy in pregnant individuals with chronic hypertension at a BP threshold of systolic BP of $\geq$ 140 mm Hg and/or diastolic BP of $\geq$ 90 mm Hg reduced the risk of poor neonatal and maternal outcomes. It is unclear if individuals with preeclampsia or gestational hypertension will derive the same maternal and neonatal benefits with the initiation of antihypertensive therapy at this same threshold.

- Much research has shown that individuals with HDPs are at higher risk of future CVD, and it is essential that clinicians elicit a pregnancy history from their patients while assessing cardiovascular risk. Currently, traditional risk factor reduction measures are recommended though there are not prospective data as to the benefit of specific risk factor reduction strategies in this population.

DISCLOSURE

The authors have nothing to disclose.

REFERENCES

1. Ford ND. Hypertensive disorders in pregnancy and mortality at delivery hospitalization — United States, 2017–2019. MMWR Morb Mortal Wkly Rep 2022;71. https://doi.org/10.15585/mmwr.mm7117a1.
2. ACOG Practice Bulletin No. 203: chronic hypertension in pregnancy. Obstet Gynecol 2019;133(1):e26.
3. Gestational hypertension and preeclampsia: ACOG Practice Bulletin, Number 222. Obstet Gynecol 2020;135(6):e237.
4. Joseph KS, Boutin A, Lisonkova S, et al. Maternal mortality in the United States: recent trends, current status, and future considerations. Obstet Gynecol 2021; 137(5):763–71.
5. Bisson C, Dautel S, Patel E, et al. Preeclampsia pathophysiology and adverse outcomes during pregnancy and postpartum. Front Med 2023;10. https://doi.org/10.3389/fmed.2023.1144170.
6. Low-dose aspirin use for the prevention of preeclampsia and related morbidity and mortality. Available at: https://www.acog.org/clinical/clinical-guidance/practice-advisory/articles/2021/12/low-dose-aspirin-use-for-the-prevention-of-preeclampsia-and-related-morbidity-and-mortality. [Accessed 14 April 2024].
7. Parikh NI, Gonzalez JM, Anderson CAM, et al. Adverse pregnancy outcomes and cardiovascular disease risk: unique opportunities for cardiovascular disease

prevention in women: a scientific statement from the American Heart Association. Circulation 2021;143(18):e902–16.

8. Rolnik DL, Wright D, Poon LC, et al. Aspirin versus placebo in pregnancies at high risk for preterm preeclampsia. N Engl J Med 2017;377(7):613–22.

9. Lin L, Huai J, Li B, et al. A randomized controlled trial of low-dose aspirin for the prevention of preeclampsia in women at high risk in China. Am J Obstet Gynecol 2022;226(2):251.e1–12.

10. Petersen TG, Liew Z, Andersen AMN, et al. Use of paracetamol, ibuprofen or aspirin in pregnancy and risk of cerebral palsy in the child. Int J Epidemiol 2018;47(1):121–30.

11. Low dose aspirin in pregnancy and early childhood development: follow up of the collaborative low dose aspirin study in pregnancy. CLASP collaborative group. Br J Obstet Gynaecol 1995;102(11):861–8.

12. ACOG Committee Opinion No. 743: Low-dose aspirin use during pregnancy. Obstet Gynecol 2018;132(1):e44–52.

13. Panagodage S, Yong HEJ, Costa FDS, et al. Low-dose acetylsalicylic acid treatment modulates the production of Cytokines and improves trophoblast function in an in vitro model of early-onset preeclampsia. Am J Pathol 2016;186(12): 3217–24.

14. Dutta S, Kumar S, Hyett J, et al. Molecular targets of aspirin and prevention of preeclampsia and their potential association with circulating extracellular vesicles during pregnancy. Int J Mol Sci 2019;20(18):4370.

15. Olson DN, Russell T, Ranzini AC. Assessment of adherence to aspirin for preeclampsia prophylaxis and reasons for nonadherence. Am J Obstet Gynecol MFM 2022;4(5). https://doi.org/10.1016/j.ajogmf.2022.100663.

16. Combs CA, Kumar NR, Morgan JL. Society for Maternal-Fetal Medicine Special Statement: Prophylactic low-dose aspirin for preeclampsia prevention—quality metric and opportunities for quality improvement. Am J Obstet Gynecol 2023; 229(2):B2–9.

17. Zhou MK, Combs CA, Pandipati S, et al. Association of checklist usage with adherence to recommended prophylactic low-dose aspirin for prevention of preeclampsia. Am J Obstet Gynecol 2023;228(3):349–51.e2.

18. Kumar NR, Speedy SE, Song J, et al. Quality improvement initiative for aspirin screening and prescription rates for preeclampsia prevention in an outpatient obstetric clinic. Am J Perinatol 2022. https://doi.org/10.1055/s-0042-1759705.

19. Rana S, Burke SD, Karumanchi SA. Imbalances in circulating angiogenic factors in the pathophysiology of preeclampsia and related disorders. Am J Obstet Gynecol 2022;226(2S):S1019–34.

20. Zeisler H, Llurba E, Chantraine F, et al. Predictive value of the sFlt-1:PlGF ratio in women with suspected preeclampsia. N Engl J Med 2016;374(1):13–22.

21. Cerdeira AS, O'Sullivan J, Ohuma EO, et al. Randomized interventional study on prediction of preeclampsia/eclampsia in women with suspected preeclampsia. Hypertension 2019;74(4):983–90.

22. Thadhani R, Lemoine E, Rana S, et al. Circulating angiogenic factor levels in hypertensive disorders of pregnancy. NEJM Evid 2022;1(12):EVIDoa2200161.

23. Schlembach D, Hund M, Schroer A, et al. Economic assessment of the use of the sFlt-1/PlGF ratio test to predict preeclampsia in Germany. BMC Health Serv Res 2018;18:603.

24. Khosla K, Espinoza J, Perlaza L, et al. Cost effectiveness of the sFlt1/PlGF ratio test as an adjunct to the current practice of evaluating suspected preeclampsia in the United States. Pregnancy Hypertens 2021;26:121–6.

25. Overview | PLGF-based testing to help diagnose suspected preterm pre-eclampsia | Guidance. NICE; 2022. Available at: https://www.nice.org.uk/guidance/dg49. [Accessed 14 April 2024].

26. Gupta S, Petras L, Tufail MU, et al. Hypertension in pregnancy: what we now know. Curr Opin Nephrol Hypertens 2023;32(2):153–64.

27. Sinkey RG, Battarbee AN, Bello NA, et al. Prevention, diagnosis, and management of hypertensive disorders of pregnancy: a comparison of international guidelines. Curr Hypertens Rep 2020;22(9):66.

28. Garovic VD, Dechend R, Easterling T, et al. Hypertension in pregnancy: diagnosis, blood pressure goals, and pharmacotherapy: a scientific statement from the American Heart Association. Hypertension 2022;79(2):e21–41.

29. von Dadelszen P, Ornstein MP, Bull SB, et al. Fall in mean arterial pressure and fetal growth restriction in pregnancy hypertension: a meta-analysis. Lancet Lond Engl 2000;355(9198):87–92.

30. Abalos E, Duley L, Steyn DW, et al. Antihypertensive drug therapy for mild to moderate hypertension during pregnancy. Cochrane Database Syst Rev 2018;10(10):CD002252.

31. Magee LA, von Dadelszen P, Evelyne R, et al. Less-tight versus tight control of hypertension in pregnancy. N Engl J Med 2015;372(5):407–17.

32. Tita AT, Szychowski JM, Boggess K, et al. Treatment for mild chronic hypertension during pregnancy. N Engl J Med 2022;386(19):1781–92.

33. Zhang Y, Liang C, Wang C, et al. Lower blood pressure achieved leads to better pregnant outcomes in non-severe chronic hypertensive pregnant women. Pregnancy Hypertens 2021;25:62–7.

34. Whelton PK, Carey RM, Aronow WS, et al. 2017 ACC/AHA/AAPA/ABC/ACPM/AGS/APhA/ASH/ASPC/NMA/PCNA Guideline for the Prevention, Detection, Evaluation, and Management of High Blood Pressure in Adults: Executive Summary: A Report of the American College of Cardiology/American Heart Association Task Force on Clinical Practice Guidelines. Hypertens Dallas Tex 1979 2018;71(6):1269–324.

35. Bone JN, Magee LA, Singer J, et al. Blood pressure thresholds in pregnancy for identifying maternal and infant risk: a secondary analysis of Community-Level Interventions for Pre-eclampsia (CLIP) trial data. Lancet Glob Health 2021;9(8):e1119–28.

36. Clinical Guidance for the integration of the findings of the chronic hypertension and pregnancy (CHAP) Study. Available at: https://www.acog.org/clinical/clinical-guidance/practice-advisory/articles/2022/04/clinical-guidance-for-the-integration-of-the-findings-of-the-chronic-hypertension-and-pregnancy-chap-study. [Accessed 14 April 2024].

37. Society for Maternal-Fetal Medicine; Publications Committee. Electronic address: pubss@mfm.org. Society for Maternal-Fetal Medicine Statement: Antihypertensive therapy for mild chronic hypertension in pregnancy-The Chronic Hypertension and Pregnancy trial. Am J Obstet Gynecol 2022;227(2):B24–7.

38. Magee LA, Brown MA, Hall DR, et al. The 2021 International Society for the Study of Hypertension in Pregnancy classification, diagnosis & management recommendations for international practice. Pregnancy Hypertens 2022;27:148–69.

39. Grandi SM, Filion KB, Yoon S, et al. Cardiovascular disease-related morbidity and mortality in women with a history of pregnancy complications. Circulation 2019;139(8):1069–79.

40. Wu R, Wang T, Gu R, et al. Hypertensive disorders of pregnancy and risk of cardiovascular disease-related morbidity and mortality: a systematic review and meta-analysis. Cardiology 2020;145(10):633–47.
41. Stuart JJ, Tanz LJ, Rimm EB, et al. Cardiovascular risk factors mediate the long-term maternal risk associated with hypertensive disorders of pregnancy. J Am Coll Cardiol 2022;79(19):1901–13.
42. Biwer LA, Lu Q, Ibarrola J, et al. Smooth muscle mineralocorticoid receptor promotes hypertension after preeclampsia. Circ Res 2023;132(6):674–89.
43. Mosca L, Benjamin EJ, Berra K, et al. Effectiveness-based guidelines for the prevention of cardiovascular disease in women–2011 update: a guideline from the American Heart Association. J Am Coll Cardiol 2011;57(12):1404–23.
44. Skurnik G, Roche AT, Stuart JJ, et al. Improving the postpartum care of women with a recent history of preeclampsia: a focus group study. Hypertens Pregnancy 2016;35(3):371–81.
45. Wilkins-Haug L, Celi A, Thomas A, et al. Recognition by Women's Health Care providers of long-term cardiovascular disease risk after preeclampsia. Obstet Gynecol 2015;125(6):1287–92.
46. Young B, Hacker MR, Rana S. Physicians' knowledge of future vascular disease in women with preeclampsia. Hypertens Pregnancy 2012;31(1):50–8.
47. Stuart JJ, Skurnik G, Roche AT, et al. Accuracy of maternal self-report of recent preeclampsia among healthy women. J Womens Health 2002. https://doi.org/10.1089/jwh.2023.0930. Published online March 29, 2024.
48. Grundy SM, Stone NJ, Bailey AL, et al. 2018 AHA/ACC/AACVPR/AAPA/ABC/ACPM/ADA/AGS/APhA/ASPC/NLA/PCNA Guideline on the Management of Blood Cholesterol: A Report of the American College of Cardiology/American Heart Association Task Force on Clinical Practice Guidelines. Circulation 2019;139(25): e1082–143.

Pregnancy in Congenital Adrenal Hyperplasia

Nicole Reisch, MD[a], Richard J. Auchus, MD, PhD[b,c],*

KEYWORDS

- Congenital adrenal hyperplasia • Pregnancy • Ovulation induction • Progesterone
- Estrogen • Glucocorticoids

KEY POINTS

- High adrenal-derived progesterone production in the follicular phase is a major impediment to conception in women with all forms of classic congenital adrenal hyperplasia (CAH) except lipoid congenital adrenal hyperplasia (LCAH).
- Women with 21-hydroxylase deficiency and 11-hydroxylase deficiency generally only require strict control of adrenal steroidogenesis to conceive, and fecundity rates are normal in properly treated patients.
- In women with 17-hydroxylase deficiency (17OHD), P450-oxidoreductase deficiency (PORD), and LCAH, the steroidogenic defect in the ovary impairs estrogen production; however, oocyte maturation can be induced with gonadotropins.
- In women with 17OHD, PORD, and LCAH, a 2-stage approach is used, with egg retrieval and embryo formation first, followed by implantation to an estrogenized uterus later.
- No cases of fertility have been described in a woman with 3β-hydroxysteroid dehydrogenase type 2 deficiency.

INTRODUCTION

Congenital adrenal hyperplasia (CAH) is a genetic (congenital) disorder of cortisol biosynthesis, which impairs the function of 1 or more enzymes or cofactor proteins needed to produce cortisol.[1] Loss of negative feedback on the hypothalamic-pituitary-adrenal (HPA) axis from the cortisol deficiency increases adrenocorticotropin (ACTH) production, even during fetal life. The tropic effect of ACTH increases the

[a] Department of Medicine IV, Institute for Endocrinology, Diabetology & Metabolism, Klinikum der Universität München, Ziemssenstraße 1, München 80336, Germany; [b] Department of Pharmacology, Division of Metabolism, Endocrinology and Diabetes, University of Michigan, MSRB II, 5560A, 1150 West Medical Center Drive, Ann Arbor, MI 48109, USA; [c] Department of Internal Medicine, Division of Metabolism, Endocrinology and Diabetes, University of Michigan, MSRB II, 5560A, 1150 West Medical Center Drive, Ann Arbor, MI 48109, USA
* Corresponding author. Division of Metabolism, Endocrinology and Diabetes, University of Michigan, MSRB II, 5560A, 1150 West Medical Center Drive, Ann Arbor, MI, 48109.
E-mail address: rauchus@med.umich.edu

Endocrinol Metab Clin N Am 53 (2024) 391–407
https://doi.org/10.1016/j.ecl.2024.05.005   endo.theclinics.com

mobilization of cholesterol for steroidogenesis and the production of precursor steroids upstream of the affected step in cortisol production. The trophic effect of ACTH stimulates growth of the adrenal cortex (adrenal hyperplasia). The pathway of cortisol biosynthesis is illustrated in **Fig. 1**, with interrelated pathways to aldosterone and 19-carbon steroids shown as well.[2] The major 19-carbon product is the sulfate conjugate of dehydroepiandrosterone (DHEA), DHEA-sulfate (DHEAS). The adrenal also produces some androstenedione, over half of which is 11β-hydroxylated to 11β-hydroxyandrostenedione, the major 19-carbon unconjugated product of the adrenal. In peripheral tissues, the 11β-hydroxyandrostenedione is metabolized to 11-ketotestosterone, a bioactive androgen with potency comparable to testosterone (**Fig. 1**).

In general, complete or nearly complete loss-of-function mutations give rise to "classic" forms of CAH, which feature clinically-manifested cortisol deficiency and can lead to adrenal crisis, particularly in infants. In contrast, "nonclassic" CAH is due to partial deficiencies, in which cortisol production is generally adequate at the expense of abnormally high precursor accumulation. The most common form of CAH is 21-hydroxylase deficiency (21OHD), due to mutations in the *CYP21A2* gene.[3] In 21OHD, some degree of androgen excess is always present, but cortisol and if complete also aldosterone deficiency occurs only in classic 21OHD. The orthogonal condition is 17-hydroxylase deficiency (17OHD), in which mutations in the *CYP17A1* gene cause androgen and estrogen deficiency with mineralocorticoid excess and, despite cortisol deficiency, glucocorticoid sufficiency due to high corticosterone production.[4] The combination of androgen and mineralocorticoid excesses in 21OHD and 17OHD occurs in 11β-hydroxylase deficiency (11OHD), due to mutations in the *CYP11B1* gene. Because 11OHD affects the last step in cortisol biosynthesis, both androgens and mineralocorticoids accumulate with the cortisol deficiency. Rare forms include P450-oxidoreductase[5] and 3β-hydroxysteroid dehydrogenase type 2[6] deficiencies (PORD and HSD3B2D, due to mutations in the *POR* and *HSD3B2* genes, respectively), which

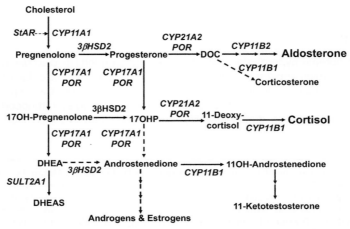

Fig. 1. Normal adrenal steroidogenic pathways to aldosterone, cortisol, and DHEAS. Subsequent metabolism of androstenedione to androgens and estrogens, as well as 11-ketotestosterone is shown for completeness. Dashed arrows indicate ordinarily minor pathways within the adrenal, such as conversion of DHEA to androstenedione in the zona reticularis or conversion of DOC to corticosterone in the zona fasciculata. *Abbreviations are as used in text, plus 17OH-Pregnenolone, 17-hydroxypregnenolone; 11OH-Androstenedione,* 11β-hydroxyandrostenedione.

feature genital ambiguity in males and females, derived from impairment of normal androgen biosynthesis pathways plus alternative pathways that often yield androgen action between normal male and female extremes. Finally, lipoid CAH (LCAH) is due to mutations in the *STAR* gene encoding the steroidogenic acute regulatory protein (StAR), which mobilizes cholesterol for steroidogenesis in the adrenal cortex and gonads.[7] In classic LCAH, all steroids are deficient, whereas only cortisol is deficient in nonclassic LCAH, because cortisol is the adrenal steroid hormone made in largest amounts ($\sim$ 500 nmol/L, 6–8 mg/m^2/d).[8] LCAH is so named because the adrenal cortex cells are laden with cholesterol esters; however, a phenocopy without cholesterol ester accumulation also exists from even more rare mutations in the *CYP11A1* gene encoding the cholesterol side-chain cleavage enzyme.[9]

In all forms of CAH, the disease is characterized by the deficient steroid hormones (in addition to cortisol), the excess steroid hormones, and the abnormal steroids that are not normally produced in significant amounts. In addition, some genes affected in the various forms of CAH are also expressed in the gonads and might directly impair steroidogenesis in the testes or ovaries (*STAR*, *CYP11A1*, *HSD3B2*, *POR*, and *CYP17A1*), whereas others are expressed only in the adrenal cortex (*CYP21A2*, *CYP11B1*). **Table 1** lists the most relevant anomalous steroid products in each form of classic CAH.

CLASSIC (SEVERE) 21-HYDROXYLASE DEFICIENCY

Women with classic 21OHD, in particular with the salt-wasting form, exhibit impaired fertility and reduced birth rates.[10–13] In the most severe salt-wasting phenotype, the fertility rate in patients with adequate vaginal opening was as low as 7% in the first report on fertility rates in classic 21OHD.[10] Owing to optimized treatment strategies and better outcomes of genital reconstruction, this low rate certainly has improved[13]; however, time to pregnancy and overall fertility is still substantially lower than in the general population. In a Swedish population-based cohort study, women with 21OHD had fewer children than controls, and only 25% of women had at least 1 child compared to 46% of the Swedish control population.[14] The reasons for this difference are multifactorial and range from hormonal imbalance to anatomic obstacles and psychosocial and psychosexual barriers. Patients with 21OHD have been found to have different gender behavior and fewer heterosexual partnerships,[15] as well as less interest in motherhood. Secondary to external genital virilization and subsequent genital surgery, patients experience barriers with vaginal intercourse and dissatisfaction with their sexual life.[15–19] Patients frequently show low satisfaction with body appearance and thus less self-confidence and sexual confidence.[18,20]

Table 1
Key biomarker steroid patterns in the congenital adrenal hyperplasia

CAH Type	Progesterone	17OHP	DOC	Corticosterone	Androgens	Estrogens
21OHD	High	High	Low	Low	High	Nl-High
11OHD	High	Nl-High	High	Low	High	Nl-High
17OHD	High	Low	High	High	Low	Low
PORD	Very High	Nl-High	Nl	Nl-High	Low	Low
LCAH	Low	Low	Low	Low	Low	Low
HSD3B2D	Nl-High	Nl-High	Low	Low	Nl-High	Low-Nl

In terms of hormonal imbalance, it is adrenal-derived progesterone and adrenal androgens combined with altered gonadotrophin secretion causing anovulation and interfering with ovulation and embryo implantation (**Fig. 2** and **Table 1**). Up to 60% of patients with classic 21OHD without contraceptive therapy report irregular menstrual cycles.[21–23] Adrenal progesterone and 17-hydroxyprogesterone (17OHP) oversecretion act like a progestin-only contraceptive pill.[24–26] The mucus in the cervix thickens, making it difficult for sperm to enter the uterus and fertilize an egg; additionally, gonadotropin secretion is suppressed, leading to anovulation. Importantly, however, it could be shown that unequal conception and pregnancy rates are primarily due to inadequate treatment and the fact that less women seek motherhood, rather than a general inability to conceive.[27] In fact, with proper treatment, those women who attempt to conceive show the same conception rates as the normal population, both in the salt-wasting and simple-virilizing phenotypes (**Box 1**). In order to stop the contraceptive effects of adrenal-derived progesterone and 17OHP as described earlier, especially progesterone secretion needs to be effectively suppressed in the follicular phase. A target of lower than 2 nmol/L (0.6 ng/mL) progesterone concentration in the follicular phase has been suggested to enable ovulation and fertilization.[27] Mostly, this goal can be achieved through an increase of glucocorticoid dosage, with the aim of suppressed progesterone and adrenal androgens at the cost of symptoms from overtreatment. Casteràs and colleagues[27] described an 8-hourly prednisolone regimen to achieve pregnancies. Additionally, increasing the fludrocortisone dose might be beneficial, as increased progesterone might also be derived from the aldosterone pathway.[28] The aim of treatment is a renin concentration in the normal range by the addition of fludrocortisone also in patients with simple-virilizing phenotype who were not taking fludrocortisone therapy prior to the desire to conceive. The impact of progesterone on pregnancy rates in 21OHD was strengthened by a study investigating luteinizing hormone (LH) pulsatility in 21OHD females, where hormonal control and in particular progesterone concentration was the best predictor of LH pulsatility.[29] The patient group with elevated progesterone and adrenal androgens showed reduced

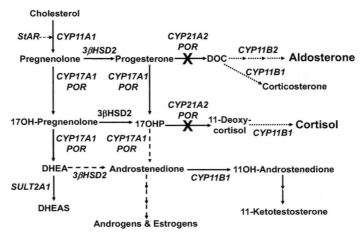

Fig. 2. Adrenal steroidogenic pathways in 21OHD. The blocks (X) in aldosterone and cortisol synthesis shunts steroidogenesis to androgens. In particular, formation of 11β-hydroxyandrostenedione and 11-ketotestosterone is increased. Depleted pathways beyond the blocks are indicated with dotted arrows. *Abbreviations are as used in text, plus 17OH-Pregnenolone, 17-hydroxypregnenolone; 11OH-Androstenedione, 11β-hydroxyandrostenedione.*

Box 1
Key issues for pregnancy in women with 21-hydroxylase deficiency

- High adrenal-derived progesterone in the follicular phase of the menstrual cycle is the major impediment to pregnancy in women with classic 21OHD.
- Fecundity rates are normal in women with classic 21OHD with proper management.
- The placenta defends the fetus from maternal androgens during pregnancy.
- Women with nonclassic 21OHD are at high risk of miscarriage, and hydrocortisone therapy from conception through pregnancy might reduce this risk.

LH pulse frequency and amplitude, which further highlights the mechanisms of anovulation in 21OHD.[29]

For glucocorticoid replacement periconceptionally and during pregnancy, only hydrocortisone or prednisolone should be administered, as both will be inactivated by placental 11β-hydroxysteroid dehydrogenase type 2 and thus will not have adverse effects on the fetus.[30] Dexamethasone, on the other hand, passes the placental barrier and thus has been used for prenatal therapy, where the effect on the fetus is wanted to prevent virilization of the external genitalia in a female fetus affected by 21OHD.[30,31] Prenatal therapy, however, is considered experimental[32] and is rarely used. In case optimal suppression of progesterone cannot be achieved by conventional hydrocortisone or prednisolone, a switch to modified-release hydrocortisone, if available, should be considered. A recent study shows that better hormonal control can be achieved, in particular during the morning, with these preparations, and the data suggest that menstrual cycles might be restored in a higher percentage than with conventional glucocorticoids.[33] Rarely, bilateral adrenalectomy has been performed in cases of severe adrenal hyperandrogenism, and successful restoration of menstrual cycles and conception have been described as outcome of the procedure.[34–37] As bilateral adrenalectomy necessitates strict patient adherence to glucocorticoid replacement and otherwise bears a high risk for both adrenal crisis and also for the development of adrenal rest tissue, this procedure is not generally recommended but should only be performed in individual cases after thoughtful consideration.

The course and outcomes of pregnancies are mostly uneventful,[38] but there are also reports on higher rates of gestational diabetes and children born small for gestational age in women with classic 21OHD.[39,40] Importantly, women with 21OHD do not seem to have a higher risk or rate of preeclampsia.[40] As a result of constricted pelvic anatomy due to genital virilization and reconstruction, women with classic 21OHD often have a higher rate of elective cesarean deliveries compared to the general population.[14,40] This elevated rate can be nearly 4 times as high as that of women without 21OHD. For individuals with the salt-wasting phenotype of 21OHD, the rate of cesarean sections can be particularly striking, reaching as high as 91% in some series.[14]

Pregnant women with 21OHD should be followed and monitored in specialized endocrine centers. Monitoring disease control during pregnancy poses a particular challenge, as all disease control markers change substantially during pregnancy, and trimester-specific reference intervals need to be applied. Steroid 17OHP increases throughout pregnancy whereas androstenedione increases by 80% until gestational week 12 and then remains constant.[41] Plasma renin concentrations (or activity) are not reliable biomarkers for optimal mineralocorticoid treatment[42] and during pregnancy even less suited as a biomarker, as concentrations normally rise.[43] Therefore, adequate mineralocorticoid and glucocorticoid replacement relies on clinical judgment, electrolytes, blood pressure, signs of volume depletion (orthostasis), blood glucose, cushingoid signs, weight gain, or hypertension. There are no specific recommendations for glucocorticoid and mineralocorticoid replacement during pregnancy. Generally, the pre-pregnancy mineralocorticoid dose remains unchanged during pregnancy, even though theoretically progesterone exerts anti-mineralocorticoid effects.[44] The gluco-corticoid dose, however, may be increased in the third trimester by 20% to 40%, as in primary adrenal insufficiency,[45] which also provides additional mineralocorticoid activity, but also this consensus is based primarily on theoretic considerations rather than the evidence-based data.

Delivery should be planned in specialized center. During labor and delivery, stress dosing is necessary with doubling or tripling the dose and a bolus of 50 to 100 mg hydrocortisone at onset of labor or prior to surgery. Depending on the duration of labor and occurrence of complications during delivery, the bolus should be followed by continuous infusion of up to 200 mg every 24 h or 50 mg every 6 h, depending on the clinical setting. Breast feeding is encouraged, as only minimal quantities of glucocorticoids are secreted into the breast milk, which poses no risk to the infant.[46]

NONCLASSIC 21-HYDROXYLASE DEFICIENCY

In nonclassic 21OHD, spontaneous pregnancy rates are high,[47–49] but increased rates of miscarriage of about 26% have been observed.[50,51] In contrast to women with classic 21OHD, females with nonclassic 21OHD have a higher desire for motherhood (50% vs 24% according to Casteràs at al.).[27] Often, nonclassic 21OHD is only diagnosed and treated after seeking medical attention for an unfulfilled wish to have children.[50,51]

Low-dose glucocorticoid replacement with hydrocortisone or prednisolone may be beneficial to achieve pregnancy and to reduce miscarriage rates.[50,51] In diabetic patients with nonclassic 21OHD, effects of metformin on reduction of 17OHP and adrenal androgens have been described.[50,51] Even though women with nonclassic 21OHD do not experience genital virilization, the rate of delivery by cesarean section is still higher than in the general population in many countries.[47] Stress dosing during pregnancy and delivery is only necessary in case of additional partial adrenal insufficiency, either endogenous or iatrogenic.

11β-HYDROXYLASE DEFICIENCY

In general, the impediments to fertility in 11OHD are the same as in 21OHD: high follicular-phase adrenal-derived progesterone, gonadotropin suppression, and vaginal inadequacy. In the chronic management of 11OHD, the hypertension is often more difficult to control with glucocorticoids than the androgen excess, and combined therapy with mineralocorticoid-receptor antagonist is often beneficial.[1] For pregnancy induction, however, a similar approach to 21OHD with progesterone suppression using divided doses of glucocorticoids is the cornerstone of therapy. Doses adequate for progesterone suppression will nearly always control both androgen and mineralocorticoid excess (**Fig. 3**). The literature contains few examples of pregnancy in women with classic 11OHD, given the rarity of the disease.[13,52] Some reports suggest that androgen excess[53] or hypertension[54] can worsen during pregnancy.

COMBINED 17-HYDROXYLASE OR 17,20-LYASE DEFICIENCY

The *CYP17A1* gene is expressed in both the adrenal cortex and gonads. Only the 17-hydroxylase activity is required for cortisol production, but both activities are

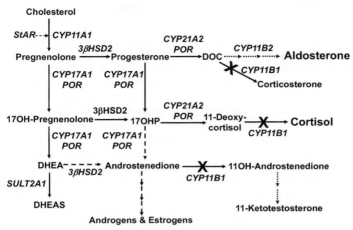

Fig. 3. Adrenal steroidogenic pathways in 11OHD. The blocks (X) in corticosterone and cortisol synthesis causes glucocorticoid deficiency, forces mineralocorticoid (DOC) accumulation, and shunts steroidogenesis to androgens. Unlike 21OHD, absence of 11β-hydroxylase activity prevents formation of 11β-hydroxyandrostenedione and 11-ketotestosterone. Aldosterone production is possible but ordinarily low due to DOC-mediated renin suppression. Depleted pathways beyond the blocks are indicated with dotted arrows. *Abbreviations are as used in text, plus 17OH-Pregnenolone, 17-hydroxypregnenolone; 11OH-Androstenedione, 11β-hydroxyandrostenedione.*

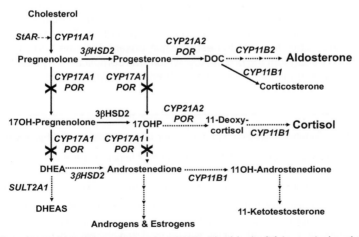

Fig. 4. Adrenal steroidogenic pathways in 17OHD. The blocks (X) in cortisol and 19-carbon steroid synthesis shunts steroidogenesis to corticosterone and forces mineralocorticoid (DOC) accumulation. Aldosterone production is possible but ordinarily low due to DOC-mediated renin suppression. The production of all androgens and estrogens is low, both in the adrenal and in the ovary. Depleted pathways beyond the blocks are indicated with dotted arrows. *Abbreviations are as used in text, plus 17OH-Pregnenolone, 17-hydroxypregnenolone; 11OH-Androstenedione, 11β-hydroxyandrostenedione.*

necessary for 19-carbon steroids production, primarily DHEA, which is a precursor for androgens and estrogens (**Fig. 4**). The sex steroid deficiency in this condition means that cyclic menses will not occur spontaneously in affected 46,XX individuals. Despite elevated gonadotropins secondary to estrogen deficiency, ovulation is infrequent, and large cystic ovaries often develop after puberty.[55] Both estrogen deficiency and adrenal-derived progesterone excess prevent development of a secretory endometrium, which lead to amenorrhea and an unreceptive uterine environment for a fertilized egg. Unlike 21OHD, progesterone suppression is insufficient to allow pregnancy, due to the estrogen deficiency and anovulation. Consequently, a multiple-step strategy must be employed (**Box 2**).

Embryos were first achieved in a woman with 17OHD using gonadotropin injections for oocyte maturation, egg retrieval, and in vitro fertilization; however, the embryo development arrested and could not lead to implantation and pregnancy.[56] Subsequently, a woman with incomplete 17OHP achieved a live birth with a phased strategy.[57] First, adrenal-derived progesterone was continuously suppressed with 0.5 mg/d dexamethasone. Next, pharmacologic menstrual bleeding was induced with oral estradiol valerate followed by micronized progesterone for 1 week and withdrawal. Endogenous gonadotropins were suppressed with leuprolide acetate starting 3 days prior to withdrawal of estrogen and progestin, and oocyte maturation was stimulated with recombinant follitropin plus estrogen. After 1 injection of chorionic gonadotropin, 4 mature eggs were retrieved and fertilized in vitro, and the developed embryos were frozen at the blastocyst stage. During gonadotropin treatment, ovary-derived progesterone will rise in women with 17OHD due to the enzymatic block in the theca cells, and this progesterone will impair endometrial lining growth, even if exogenous estrogen is supplied. Therefore, implantation must be delayed until endometrial preparation can be achieved pharmacologically.

One month subsequently, depot goserelin acetate was administered, and 3 months later, the serum progesterone was adequately suppressed at 0.6 ng/mL, and uterine preparation commenced with estradiol valerate for 28 days. During the last 5 days, micronized progesterone was added, and 2 embryos were implanted. Ultrasound confirmed a singleton pregnancy at 6 weeks of gestation. Estradiol was tapered and discontinued after the first trimester, while dexamethasone and progesterone were continued throughout the pregnancy, which was complicated by gestational diabetes, cholestasis gravidarum, a lower extremity cellulitis, and pre-eclampsia. A

Box 2
Key issues for pregnancy in women with rare forms of congenital adrenal hyperplasia

- In 17OHD, PORD, and LCAH, the defect in the adrenal impairs cortisol production, and the same defect in the ovary impairs estradiol production in the developing follicles.

- Gonadotropins can induce oocyte maturation even with negligible estradiol production.

- A two-stage approach is typically used in these women, unlike women with 21OHD.

- The first phase involves adrenal-derived progesterone suppression in 17OHD and PORD, oocyte maturation with gonadotropins, egg retrieval, and embryo generation with in vitro fertilization, which are frozen for later use.

- The second phase involves adrenal-derived progesterone suppression in 17OHD and PORD, uterine preparation with sequential estradiol and progesterone, and implantation of thawed embryos.

- Women with LCAH require progesterone supplementation until the luteo-placental shift.

healthy male infant was delivered via caesarean section at 30 weeks' gestation for fetal distress.[57]

A few additional case reports have described pregnancy in women with 17OHD.[58] Common themes have emerged from these studies include: most cases are incomplete, combined 17-hydroxylase or 17,20-lyase deficiency or in 1 case isolated (preferential) 17,20-lyase deficiency; the importance of suppressing adrenal and ovarian progesterone production; oocyte maturation and harvesting to form embryos first, followed by uterine preparation and implantation of stored embryos. Because the ovary is also 17-hydroxylase deficient, ovarian-derived progesterone rises during gonadotropin stimulation as well; consequently, adequate growth of the uterine lining will not occur simultaneously, even if exogenous estrogen is supplied. Thus, unlike 21OHD or 11OHD, women with 17OHD must receive disease-specific treatment for disordered steroidogenesis with progesterone accumulation in both the adrenal and ovary. Whether pregnancy can be achieved in complete, combined 17-hydroxylase or 17,20-lyase deficiency remains unknown.

Because so few examples of pregnancy in 17OHD have been described, the optimal management strategy during pregnancy is not known. In theory, no treatment is needed after the luteo-placental shift by the tenth week of gestation. First, the steroidogenic component of the placenta (syncitiotrophoblast) is fetal tissue capable of making progesterone and of converting DHEAS derived from the fetal adrenal to estrogens.[59] Second, corticosterone from the maternal adrenal prevents glucocorticoid deficiency in both mother and fetus. It is not possible to distinguish whether the pregnancy complications described in the case of Bianchi and colleagues were due to continued dexamethasone, intrinsic to the maternal milieu, or both.

P450-OXIDOREDUCTASE DEFICIENCY

Conceptually, PORD is a variably incomplete combination of 21OHD and 17OHD, with the added non-adrenal impairment of aromatase (P450 19A1) activity needed for estrogen production (**Fig. 5**). For individual patients, however, the specific *POR* missense mutations with incomplete loss of function typically influence the various microsomal (type 2) cytochrome P450 activities in unique profiles, leading to dissimilar degrees of impairment in the various steroid hydroxylase activities.[60,61] For example, the A287P mutation, which is common in Caucasians, impairs 17-hydroxylase activity by greater than 50% and more than 21-hydroxylase activity but affords normal aromatase activity. In contrast, mutation R457H, which is common in Japan and Korea, eliminates nearly all aromatase and 17-hydroxylase activities, thus resembling 17OHD more than mutation A287P. The rare G539R mutation affords a phenocopy of isolated 17,20-lyase deficiency.[62] As in 17OHD, PORD impairs both adrenal and ovarian steroidogenesis, and reproductive strategies must address the specific problems in both organs. Given that the aberrant steroidogenesis in the ovary creates additional reproductive challenges,[63] the approach to pregnancy in PORD resembles that used in 17OHD, rather than simply suppression of adrenal-derived progesterone as in 21OHD and 11OHD.

Analogous to the process used in women with 17OHD, adrenal-derived progesterone suppression with dexamethasone, ovulation induction with follitropin followed by chorionic gonadotropin, and egg retrieval has led to successful embryo formation using in vitro fertilization.[64–67] Because, as in 17OHD, progesterone rises during ovarian stimulation for women with PORD, uterine preparation must follow egg retrieval and in vitro fertilization. In one case, dexamethasone was discontinued after implantation of 2 embryos, with estrogen and progesterone support during the first trimester.[64] No

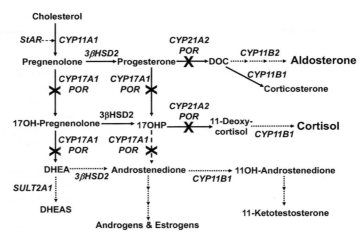

Fig. 5. Adrenal steroidogenic pathways in PORD. The variable blocks (X) in aldosterone, cortisol and 19-carbon steroid synthesis causes marked accumulation of progesterone in the adrenal and ovary. Both 17OHP and corticosterone, which are downstream of one block, can be normal or high. Cortisol, androgens, and estrogens, which are downstream of 2 or 3 blocks, are typically low but not absent. Aldosterone production is possible but has not been studied in detail. Depleted pathways beyond the blocks are indicated with dotted arrows. *Abbreviations are as used in text, plus 17OH-Pregnenolone, 17-hydroxypregnenolone; 11OH-Androstenedione,* 11β-hydroxyandrostenedione.

complications or clinical adrenal insufficiency developed during this pregnancy, and 2 healthy fraternal twin babies were delivered via caesarean section at 37 weeks of gestation. This case suggests that, if clinically adrenal insufficiency is not manifest prior to pregnancy and pre-pregnancy treatment has not caused HPA axis suppression, glucocorticoids can be discontinued in women with PORD during pregnancy, with tapering and serial testing if HPA axis status is unclear. Curiously, the common A287P and R457H mutations are poorly represented in these women who have achieved pregnancies,[64] which might imply that milder and less common mutations are more likely to portend success with assisted reproduction.

LIPOID CONGENITAL ADRENAL HYPERPLASIA

In LCAH, all steroidogenesis is impaired; therefore, uniquely among the forms of CAH, progesterone does not accumulate in LCAH (**Fig. 6**), and neither ACTH nor gonadotropin suppression is important for fertility. As in 17OHD and POR deficiencies, estrogen deficiency impairs uterine development prior to implantation. The idea that pregnancy could be achieved in LCAH was met with great skepticism, given the assumption that ovarian estrogen production is necessary for ovulation, but the success achieved in women with 17OHD argued that gonadotropins rather than endogenous estradiol synthesis was the primary driver of oocyte maturation and ovulation. Because the ovaries do not make significant steroids in utero, the toxicity of cholesterol ester accumulation does not occur as in the adrenal cortex and Leydig cells during fetal life, and pubertal girls with often have some breast development and even spontaneous menses, at least for a several cycles.[7,68]

Nevertheless, oocyte maturation, in vitro fertilization, and subsequent embryo implantation to a uterus prepared with exogenous estrogen and progesterone has led to successful pregnancies in women with LCAH.[69,70] These cases are similar to the

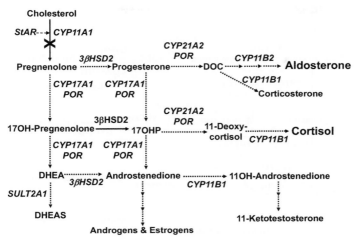

Fig. 6. Adrenal steroidogenic pathways in LCAH. The block (X) in conversion of cholesterol to pregnenolone reduces production of all steroids and prevents progesterone accumulation. Depleted pathways beyond the block are indicated with dotted arrows. *Abbreviations are as used in text, plus 17OH-Pregnenolone, 17-hydroxypregnenolone; 11OH-Androstenedione,* 11β-hydroxyandrostenedione.

protocol used for 17OHD and PORD, yet without need for glucocorticoid suppression of adrenal-derived progesterone, and progesterone supplementation was used in the first trimester (see **Box 2**). In addition, clomiphene-induced ovulation with progesterone supplementation has resulted in pregnancies for women with classic LCAH and pubertal progression.[71,72] This woman with LCAH has had 3 pregnancies, 1 without treatment that spontaneously terminated, and 2 with clomiphene that resulted in 3 children. Remarkably, her homozygous L275P mutations in the *STAR* gene produce a completely non-functional protein in vitro. It is not known whether other modifier genes or StAR-independent steroidogenesis facilitated these remarkable pregnancies in this woman.

Because the fetus is only a carrier for LCAH, both DHEAS production from the fetal adrenal and placental steroidogenesis are normal in pregnancies for women affected with LCAH, including estrogen and progesterone production after the luteo-placental shift during the first trimester. Nevertheless, because the mother has no adrenal steroid production, replacement hydrocortisone and fludrocortisone must be continued throughout pregnancy as in any woman with primary adrenal insufficiency.

3β-HYDROXYSTEROID DEHYDROGENASE TYPE 2 DEFICIENCY

In HSD3B2D, the defect impairs conversion of 3β-hydroxy-Δ⁵-steroids to their 3-keto-Δ⁴-congeners in both the adrenals and gonads. Because the type 1 isoenzyme remains normal and is expressed in skin and liver, much of these abundant adrenal-derived Δ⁵-steroids are converted 1 step further to Δ⁴-intermediates such as progesterone, 17OHP, and androstenedione (**Fig. 7**).[73] Newborn girls have moderate androgen excess but limited genital virilization, while boys are undervirilized, similar to PORD.[6] Some peripheral conversion to estrogen occurs, but menses and ovulation are generally erratic, especially in a milieu of constantly elevated adrenal-derived progesterone. No examples of pregnancy in women with classic HSD3B2D could be found in the literature. If an affected woman was attempting to conceive, the approach

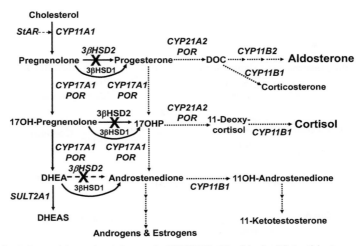

Fig. 7. Adrenal steroidogenic pathways in HSD3B2D. The blocks (X) in aldosterone, cortisol, and conversion of DHEA to androgens and estrogens cause the accumulation of inactive 3β-hydroxy-Δ⁵-steroids. The presence of the type 1 isoenzyme enables conversion of these precursors to the 3-keto-Δ⁴-steroids progesterone, 17OHP, and androstenedione in peripheral tissues, but these steroids do not re-enter the adrenals and ovary for further metabolism to a significant extent. Depleted pathways beyond the blocks are indicated with dotted arrows. *Abbreviations are as used in text, plus 17OH-Pregnenolone, 17-hydroxypregnenolone; 11OH-Androstenedione,* 11β-hydroxyandrostenedione.

would likely require both adrenal-derived progesterone suppression and estrogen supplementation for uterine lining development, possibly also with ovulation induction. Thus, the protocol would likely resemble the 2-stage approach used in 17OHD and PORD, rather than simply aggressive disease control as used in 21OHD.

SUMMARY

In women with all forms of classic CAH except LCAH, adrenal-derived follicular-phase progesterone is a major impediment to conception, primarily through impairing the development of a receptive uterine lining in the follicular phase. Progesterone also promotes unfavorable cervical mucus properties for sperm penetration and interferes with optimal gonadotropin pulsatility. In 17OHD, PORD, LCAH, and HSD3B2D, the steroidogenic defect is also present in the ovaries, which impairs estrogen production even when disease control is adequate and progesterone is well suppressed. Thus, women with 21OHD and 11OHD generally only require strict control of adrenal steroidogenesis to conceive. In contrast, women with 17OHD, PORD, LCAH, and probably HSD3B2D typically require a 2-stage protocol that involves egg retrieval with embryo generation and freezing, and then embryo implantation to a properly estrogenized uterine cavity. From these rare genetic disorders, the field has learned that ovarian estrogen production is not strictly required for ovulation in humans. The remarkable achievements of live births in these few women are superb examples of the application of science and a deep understanding of the interplay between the adrenal, ovary, pituitary, and uterus to assisted reproductive techniques.

CLINICS CARE POINTS

- For women with classic 21-hydroxylase deficiency, adrenal-derived progesterone suppression in the follicular phase is the key to achieving pregnancy.
- For women with nonclassic 21-hydroxylase deficiency, the risk of miscarriage is high and might be reduced with hydrocortisone therapy.
- Women with forms of CAH that impair both adrenal and ovarian steroidogenesis require a 2-stage process, with ovulation induction to form embryos, followed by implantation of thawed embryos after uterine preparation.

DISCLOSURE

R.J. Auchus reports contracted research support and consulting fees from Neurocrine Biosciences, Diurnal LTD, and Crinetics Pharmaceuticals; contracted research support from Spruce Biosciences; and consulting fees from H Lundbeck A/S, Novo Nordisk, and OMass Therapeutics. N. Reisch reports consulting fees from Spruce Biosciences, Neurocrine Biosciences, United States, Diurnal LTD, and H Lundbeck A/S.

FUNDING

This work was supported by the Deutsche Forschungsgemeinschaft, Germany (Heisenberg Professorship 325,768,017 to NR and Projektnummer: 314061271-TRR 205 to NR).

ACKNOWLEDGMENTS

None.

REFERENCES

1. Auchus RJ. The classic and nonclassic concenital adrenal hyperplasias. Endocr Pract 2015;21(4):383–9.
2. Miller WL, Auchus RJ. The molecular biology, biochemistry, and physiology of human steroidogenesis and its disorders. Endocr Rev 2011;32:81–151.
3. Claahsen-van der Grinten HL, Speiser PW, Ahmed SF, et al. Congenital adrenal hyperplasia-current insights in pathophysiology, diagnostics, and management. Endocr Rev 2022;43(1):91–159.
4. Auchus RJ. Steroid 17-hydroxylase and 17,20-lyase deficiencies, genetic and pharmacologic. J Steroid Biochem Mol Biol 2017;165(Pt A):71–8.
5. Huang N, Pandey AV, Agrawal V, et al. Diversity and function of mutations in P450 oxidoreductase in patients with Antley-Bixler syndrome and disordered steroidogenesis. Am J Hum Genet 2005;76:729–49.
6. Moisan AM, Ricketts ML, Tardy V, et al. New insight into the molecular basis of 3β-hydroxysteroid dehydrogenase deficiency: Identification of eight mutations in the *HSD3B2* gene in eleven patients from seven new families and comparison of the functional properties of twenty-five mutant enzymes. J Clin Endocrinol Metab 1999;84(12):4410–25.
7. Bose HS, Sugawara T, Strauss JF III, et al. The pathophysiology and genetics of congenital lipoid adrenal hyperplasia. N Engl J Med 1996;335:1870–8.
8. Baker BY, Lin L, Kim CJ, et al. Nonclassic congenital lipoid adrenal hyperplasia: A new disorder of the steroidogenic acute regulatory protein with very late presentation and normal male genitalia. J Clin Endocrinol Metab 2006;91(12):4781–5.

9. Tajima T, Fujieda K, Kouda N, et al. Heterozygous mutation in the cholesterol side chain cleavage enzyme (P450scc) gene in a patient with 46,XY sex reversal and adrenal insufficiency. J Clin Endocrinol Metab 2001;86(8):3820–5.

10. Mulaikal RM, Migeon CJ, Rock JA. Fertility rates in female patients with congenital adrenal hyperplasia due to 21-hydroxylase deficiency. N Engl J Med 1987;316: 178–82.

11. Gastaud F, Bouvattier C, Duranteau L, et al. Impaired sexual and reproductive outcomes in women with classical forms of congenital adrenal hyperplasia. J Clin Endocrinol Metab 2007;92(4):1391–6.

12. Slowikowska-Hilczer J, Hirschberg AL, Claahsen-van der Grinten H, et al. Fertility outcome and information on fertility issues in individuals with different forms of disorders of sex development: Findings from the dsd-LIFE study. Fertil Steril 2017;108(5):822–31.

13. Reisch N. Pregnancy in congenital adrenal hyperplasia. Endocrinol Metab Clin N Am 2019;48(3):619–41.

14. Hirschberg AL, Gidlof S, Falhammar H, et al. Reproductive and perinatal outcomes in women with congenital adrenal hyperplasia: A population-based cohort study. J Clin Endocrinol Metab 2021;106(2):e957–65.

15. Meyer-Bahlburg HF, Dolezal C, Baker SW, et al. Sexual orientation in women with classical or non-classical congenital adrenal hyperplasia as a function of degree of prenatal androgen excess. Arch Sex Behav 2008;37(1):85–99.

16. Almasri J, Zaiem F, Rodriguez-Gutierrez R, et al. Genital reconstructive surgery in females with congenital adrenal hyperplasia: A systematic review and meta-analysis. J Clin Endocrinol Metab 2018;103(11):4089–96.

17. Krege S, Walz KH, Hauffa BP, et al. Long-term follow-up of female patients with congenital adrenal hyperplasia from 21-hydroxylase deficiency, with special emphasis on the results of vaginoplasty. BJU Int 2000;86(3):253–8 [discussion 258-259].

18. Nordenstrom A, Frisen L, Falhammar H, et al. Sexual function and surgical outcome in women with congenital adrenal hyperplasia due to CYP21A2 deficiency: Clinical perspective and the patients' perception. J Clin Endocrinol Metab 2010;95(8):3633–40.

19. Sircili MH, Bachega TS, Madureira G, et al. Surgical treatment after failed primary correction of urogenital sinus in female patients with virilizing congenital adrenal hyperplasia: Are good results possible? Front Pediatr 2016;4:118.

20. Tschaidse L, Quinkler M, Claahsen-van der Grinten H, et al. Body image and quality of life in women with congenital adrenal hyperplasia. J Clin Med 2022; 11(15).

21. Richards GE, Grumbach MM, Kaplan SL, et al. The effect of long acting glucocorticoids on menstrual abnormalities in patients with virilizing congenital adrenal hyperplasia. J Clin Endocrinol Metab 1978;47(6):1208–15.

22. Stikkelbroeck NM, Sweep CG, Braat DD, et al. Monitoring of menstrual cycles, ovulation, and adrenal suppression by saliva sampling in female patients with 21-hydroxylase deficiency. Fertil Steril 2003;80(4):1030–6.

23. Turcu AF, Mallappa A, Elman MS, et al. 11-Oxygenated androgens are biomarkers of adrenal volume and testicular adrenal rest tumors in 21-hydroxylase deficiency. J Clin Endocrinol Metab 2017;102(8):2701–10.

24. Holmes-Walker DJ, Conway GS, Honour JW, et al. Menstrual disturbance and hypersecretion of progesterone in women with congenital adrenal hyperplasia due to 21-hydroxylase deficiency. Clin Endocrinol (Oxf) 1995;43(3):291–6.

25. Labarta E, Martinez-Conejero JA, Alama P, et al. Endometrial receptivity is affected in women with high circulating progesterone levels at the end of the follicular phase: A functional genomics analysis. Hum Reprod 2011;26(7):1813–25.
26. Mnif MF, Kamoun M, Kacem FH, et al. Reproductive outcomes of female patients with congenital adrenal hyperplasia due to 21-hydroxylase deficiency. Indian J Endocrinol Metab 2013;17(5):790–3.
27. Casteràs A, De Silva P, Rumsby G, et al. Reassessing fecundity in women with classical congenital adrenal hyperplasia (CAH): Normal pregnancy rate but reduced fertility rate. Clin Endocrinol (Oxf) 2009;70:833–7.
28. Hoepffner W, Schulze E, Bennek J, et al. Pregnancies in patients with congenital adrenal hyperplasia with complete or almost complete impairment of 21-hydroxylase activity. Fertil Steril 2004;81(5):1314–21.
29. Bachelot A, Chakhtoura Z, Plu-Bureau G, et al. Influence of hormonal control on lh pulsatility and secretion in women with classical congenital adrenal hyperplasia. Eur J Endocrinol 2012;167(4):499–505.
30. Auer MK, Nordenstrom A, Lajic S, et al. Congenital adrenal hyperplasia. Lancet 2023;401(10372):227–44.
31. Van't Westeinde A, Karlsson L, Messina V, et al. An update on the long-term outcomes of prenatal dexamethasone treatment in congenital adrenal hyperplasia. Endocr Connect 2023;12(4).
32. Speiser PW, Arlt W, Auchus RJ, et al. Congenital adrenal hyperplasia due to steroid 21-hydroxylase deficiency: An Endocrine Society clinical practice guideline. J Clin Endocrinol Metab 2018;103(11):4043–88.
33. Merke DP, Mallappa A, Arlt W, et al. Modified-release hydrocortisone in congenital adrenal hyperplasia. J Clin Endocrinol Metab 2021;106(5):e2063–77.
34. Ogilvie CM, Rumsby G, Kurzawinski T, et al. Outcome of bilateral adrenalectomy in congenital adrenal hyperplasia: One unit's experience. Eur J Endocrinol 2006; 154(3):405–8.
35. Van Wyk JJ, Ritzen EM. The role of bilateral adrenalectomy in the treatment of congenital adrenal hyperplasia. J Clin Endocrinol Metab 2003;88(7):2993–8.
36. Dagalakis U, Mallappa A, Elman M, et al. Positive fertility outcomes in a female with classic congenital adrenal hyperplasia following bilateral adrenalectomy. Int J Pediatr Endocrinol 2016;2016:10.
37. MacKay D, Nordenstrom A, Falhammar H. Bilateral adrenalectomy in congenital adrenal hyperplasia: A systematic review and meta-analysis. J Clin Endocrinol Metab 2018;103(5):1767–78.
38. Krone N, Wachter I, Stefanidou M, et al. Mothers with congenital adrenal hyperplasia and their children: Outcome of pregnancy, birth and childhood. Clin Endocrinol (Oxf) 2001;55(4):523–9.
39. Bosdou JK, Anagnostis P, Goulis DG, et al. Risk of gestational diabetes mellitus in women achieving singleton pregnancy spontaneously or after art: A systematic review and meta-analysis. Hum Reprod Update 2020;26(4):514–44.
40. Guo X, Zhang Y, Yu Y, et al. Getting pregnant with congenital adrenal hyperplasia: Assisted reproduction and pregnancy complications. A systematic review and meta-analysis. Front Endocrinol (Lausanne) 2022;13:982953.
41. Soldin OP, Guo T, Weiderpass E, et al. Steroid hormone levels in pregnancy and 1 year postpartum using isotope dilution tandem mass spectrometry. Fertil Steril 2005;84(3):701–10.
42. Pofi R, Prete A, Thornton-Jones V, et al. Plasma renin measurements are unrelated to mineralocorticoid replacement dose in patients with primary adrenal insufficiency. J Clin Endocrinol Metab 2020;105(1).

43. Hsueh WA, Luetscher JA, Carlson EJ, et al. Changes in active and inactive renin throughout pregnancy. J Clin Endocrinol Metab 1982;54(5):1010–6.
44. Quinkler M, Meyer B, Oelkers W, et al. Renal inactivation, mineralocorticoid generation, and 11β-hydroxysteroid dehydrogenase inhibition ameliorate the antimineralocorticoid effect of progesterone in vivo. J Clin Endocrinol Metab 2003; 88(8):3767–72.
45. Bornstein SR, Allolio B, Arlt W, et al. Diagnosis and treatment of primary adrenal insufficiency: An Endocrine Society clinical practice guideline. J Clin Endocrinol Metab 2016;101(2):364–89.
46. McKenzie SA, Selley JA, Agnew JE. Secretion of prednisolone into breast milk. Arch Dis Child 1975;50(11):894–6.
47. Eyal O, Ayalon-Dangur I, Segev-Becker A, et al. Pregnancy in women with non-classic congenital adrenal hyperplasia: Time to conceive and outcome. Clin Endocrinol (Oxf) 2017;87(5):552–6.
48. Nordenstrom A, Falhammar H. Management of endocrine disease: Diagnosis and management of the patient with non-classic CAH due to 21-hydroxylase deficiency. Eur J Endocrinol 2019;180(3):R127–45.
49. Carrière C, Nguyen LS, Courtillot C, et al. Fertility and pregnancy outcomes in women with nonclassic 21-hydroxylase deficiency. Clin Endocrinol (Oxf) 2023; 98(3):315–22.
50. Bidet M, Bellanne-Chantelot C, Galand-Portier MB, et al. Fertility in women with nonclassical congenital adrenal hyperplasia due to 21-hydroxylase deficiency. J Clin Endocrinol Metab 2010;95(3):1182–90.
51. Moran C, Azziz R, Weintrob N, et al. Reproductive outcome of women with 21-hydroxylase-deficient nonclassic adrenal hyperplasia. J Clin Endocrinol Metab 2006;91(9):3451–6.
52. Gomes LG, Bachega T, Mendonca BB. Classic congenital adrenal hyperplasia and its impact on reproduction. Fertil Steril 2019;111(1):7–12.
53. Simm PJ, Zacharin MR. Successful pregnancy in a patient with severe 11-beta-hydroxylase deficiency and novel mutations in CYP11B1 gene. Horm Res 2007;68(6):294–7.
54. Krishnan K, Pillai S, Vaidyanathan G. Pregnancy in a woman with congenital adrenal hyperplasia with 11-beta-hydroxylase deficiency: A case report. Obstet Med 2023;16(1):66–8.
55. ten Kate-Booij MJ, Cobbaert C, Koper JW, et al. Deficiency of 17,20-lyase causing giant ovarian cysts in a girl and a female phenotype in her 46,XY sister: Case report. Hum Reprod 2004;19(2):456–9.
56. Rabinovici J, Blankstein J, Goldman B, et al. In vitro fertilization and primary embryonic cleavage are possible in 17α-hydroxylase deficiency despite extremely low intrafollicular 17β-estradiol. J Clin Endocrinol Metab 1989;68(3):693–7.
57. Bianchi PH, Gouveia GR, Costa EM, et al. Successful live birth in a woman with 17α-hydroxylase deficiency through IVF frozen-thawed embryo transfer. J Clin Endocrinol Metab 2016;101(2):345–8.
58. van Oosbree A, Asif A, Hmaidan S, et al. Pregnancy outcomes in in vitro fertilization in 17-alpha-hydroxylase deficiency. F S Rep 2023;4(2):144–9.
59. Miller WL. Steroid hormone biosynthesis and actions in the materno-feto-placental unit. Clin Perinatol 1998;25:799–817.
60. Burkhard FZ, Parween S, Udhane SS, et al. P450 oxidoreductase deficiency: Analysis of mutations and polymorphisms. J Steroid Biochem Mol Biol 2017; 165(Pt A):38–50.

61. Huang N, Agrawal V, Giacomini KM, et al. Genetics of P450 oxidoreductase: Sequence variation in 842 individuals of four ethnicities and activities of 15 missense mutations. Proc Natl Acad Sci U S A 2008;105(5):1733–8.
62. Hershkovitz E, Parvari R, Wudy SA, et al. Homozygous mutation G539R in the gene for P450 oxidoreductase in a family previously diagnosed as having 17,20-lyase deficiency. J Clin Endocrinol Metab 2008;93(9):3584–8.
63. Gusmano C, Cannarella R, Crafa A, et al. Congenital adrenal hyperplasia, disorders of sex development, and infertility in patients with *POR* gene pathogenic variants: A systematic review of the literature. J Endocrinol Invest 2023;46(1):1–14.
64. Pan P, Zheng L, Chen X, et al. Successful live birth in a chinese woman with P450 oxidoreductase deficiency through frozen-thawed embryo transfer: A case report with review of the literature. J Ovarian Res 2021;14(1):22.
65. Papadakis GE, Dumont A, Bouligand J, et al. Non-classic cytochrome P450 oxidoreductase deficiency strongly linked with menstrual cycle disorders and female infertility as primary manifestations. Hum Reprod 2020;35(4):939–49.
66. Song T, Wang B, Chen H, et al. In vitro fertilization-frozen embryo transfer in a patient with cytochrome P450 oxidoreductase deficiency: A case report. Gynecol Endocrinol 2018;34(5):385–8.
67. Zhang T, Li Z, Ren X, et al. Clinical and genetic analysis of cytochrome P450 oxidoreductase (POR) deficiency in a female and the analysis of a novel POR intron mutation causing alternative mRNA splicing : Overall analysis of a female with POR deficiency. J Assist Reprod Genet 2020;37(10):2503–11.
68. Bose HS, Pescovitz OH, Miller WL. Spontaneous feminization in a 46,XX female patient with congenital lipoid adrenal hyperplasia caused by a homozygous frame-shift mutation in the steroidogenic acute regulatory protein. J Clin Endocrinol Metab 1997;82:1511–5.
69. Albarel F, Perrin J, Jegaden M, et al. Successful IVF pregnancy despite inadequate ovarian steroidogenesis due to congenital lipoid adrenal hyperplasia (CLAH): A case report. Hum Reprod 2016;31(11):2609–12.
70. Sertedaki A, Pantos K, Vrettou C, et al. Conception and pregnancy outcome in a patient with 11-bp deletion of the steroidogenic acute regulatory protein gene. Fertil Steril 2009;91(3):934.e915–8.
71. Khoury K, Barbar E, Ainmelk Y, et al. Thirty-eight-year follow-up of two sibling lipoid congenital adrenal hyperplasia patients due to homozygous steroidogenic acute regulatory (STARD1) protein mutation. Molecular structure and modeling of the STARD1 L275P mutation. Front Neurosci 2016;10:527.
72. Khoury K, Barbar E, Ainmelk Y, et al. Gonadal function, first cases of pregnancy, and child delivery in a woman with lipoid congenital adrenal hyperplasia. J Clin Endocrinol Metab 2009;94(4):1333–7.
73. Auchus RJ. The uncommon forms of congenital adrenal hyperplasia. Curr Opin Endocrinol Diabetes Obes 2022;29(3):263–70.

Prolactinomas
Preconception and During Pregnancy

Catherine D. Zhang, MD[a], Adriana G. Ioachimescu, MD, PhD[a,b],*

KEYWORDS

- Prolactinoma • Hyperprolactinemia • Fertility • Preconception • Pregnancy
- Apoplexy

KEY POINTS

- Premenopausal women with prolactinomas often present with hypogonadism and infertility.
- Dopamine agonists (DAs) are effective at restoring ovulation and fertility in most women. Surgery before pregnancy is considered for cases of DA intolerance or resistance.
- Short term exposure to bromocriptine and cabergoline during early pregnancy is not associated with elevated risk for adverse maternal or fetal outcomes.
- The risk of symptomatic tumor growth during pregnancy depends on pre-pregnancy tumor size and prior treatment, including duration of DA therapy.
- Spontaneous remission of prolactinomas may occur after pregnancy.

INTRODUCTION

Prolactinomas—pituitary adenomas (PAs) derived from lactotrophs—are the most common type of pituitary tumor in clinical practice. They represent 40% to 60% of all PAs and nearly 80% of functioning PAs with an estimated incidence of 2 to 8.2 new cases per 100,000/y.[1,2] Prolactinomas predominantly affect women between the ages of 25 and 44 years with important implications for fertility and pregnancy.[1,2] In this review, we discuss the clinical outcomes and approach to the management of women with prolactinomas preconception, during pregnancy, and postpartum.

FERTILITY

Premenopausal women typically present with microprolactinomas (microprolactinoma to macroprolactinoma ratio of 8:1) and oligo/amenorrhea, galactorrhea, and

[a] Department of Medicine, Division of Endocrinology and Molecular Medicine, Medical College of Wisconsin, HUB for Collaborative Medicine, 8701 Watertown Plank Road, Milwaukee, WI 53226, USA; [b] Department of Neurosurgery, Medical College of Wisconsin, HUB for Collaborative Medicine, 8701 Watertown Plank Road, Milwaukee, WI 53226, USA
* Corresponding author.
E-mail address: aioachimescu@mcw.edu

Endocrinol Metab Clin N Am 53 (2024) 409–419
https://doi.org/10.1016/j.ecl.2024.05.004
endo.theclinics.com
0889-8529/24/© 2024 Elsevier Inc. All rights reserved, including those for text and data mining, AI training, and similar technologies.

infertility rather than mass effect symptoms.[2–4] In women seeking evaluation for infertility, the prevalence of hyperprolactinemia is at least 10 fold higher than that in the general population, occurring in 5% to 7% of asymptomatic women and 33% of women with oligo/amenorrhea and/or galactorrhea.[5–8]

Pathophysiology

Hyperprolactinemia causes decreased fertility via its effects on the hypothalamic-pituitary-gonadal axis at both the central and the peripheral level (**Box 1**). At the central level, the main mechanism of prolactin-induced hypogonadism is inhibition of hypothalamic kisspeptin secretion leading to impaired gonadotropin-releasing hormone pulsatility.[9–11] Hyperprolactinemia can also directly suppress gonadotropin secretion via loss of the positive estradiol feedback on gonadotropin release at midcycle.[12] Large macroprolactinomas may cause mass effect and other pituitary hormones deficiencies that can additionally impact fertility.

At the peripheral level, hyperprolactinemia impairs estrogen and progesterone production from the ovaries. Prolactin receptors are expressed by ovarian granulosa cells, and while prolactin at low concentrations is necessary for normal sex hormone production, higher concentrations of prolactin can inhibit basal and gonadotropin-stimulated progesterone production.[13,14] This can lead to a shortened luteal phase. Adequate progesterone levels are necessary for endometrium proliferation and embryo implantation, and infertility can be observed in women with mild hyperprolactinemia and regular menses.[15,16]

Preconception Treatment Outcomes

Dopamine agonists (DAs) are effective at inducing ovulation and fertility and remain the first choice of therapy in most women with prolactinomas who desire pregnancy.[2,17] In the Webster and colleagues landmark study of 459 women with hyperprolactinemic amenorrhea (including 279 microprolactinomas and 3 macroprolactinomas), normalization of prolactin levels was achieved in 83% of women on cabergoline (0.5–2.0 mg total/wk) and 59% of women on bromocriptine (2.5–10 mg total/d). Cabergoline was more effective than bromocriptine at inducing pregnancy (72% and 52%, respectively) and had lower rates of treatment discontinuation due to side effects.[18] In another study of women with prolactinomas (29 macroprolactinomas and 56 microprolactinomas) desiring pregnancy, ovulation was achieved in 100% and pregnancy in 94% of patients treated with cabergoline.[19] Women who are not interested in fertility should be advised to use contraception when starting DAs, because return of fertility can occur before the resumption of menses.

Box 1
Effects of prolactin on the reproductive axis and fertility in women

Central mechanisms:
- Suppression of pulsatile gonadotropin-releasing hormone secretion via inhibition of hypothalamic kisspeptin.
- Loss of the positive feedback of estradiol on midcycle gonadotropin release.
- Pituitary hormone deficiencies due to compression of the pituitary gland by large prolactinomas.

Peripheral mechanisms:
- Suppression of baseline and gonadotropin-stimulated estrogen and progesterone synthesis from the ovaries.
- Shortened luteal phase due to decreased progesterone concentration.

Surgical treatment with transsphenoidal resection can normalize prolactin and restore fertility but may be less effective than DAs and requires neurosurgical expertise. Thus, surgery is typically reserved for those with DA resistance/intolerance and/or patient preference.[2] Better outcomes are observed with surgery in women with microprolactinomas. In a systematic review and meta-analysis of clinical outcomes after transsphenoidal surgery (25 studies, 1836 patients), normoprolactinemia was achieved in 83% of patients with microprolactinomas versus 60% of patients with macroprolactinomas. Postoperative hypopituitarism was reported in only 2% of patients.[20] In a surgical series focused on women of reproductive age (n = 99), prolactin levels normalized in 81% of microprolactinomas and 52% of macroprolactinomas following transsphenoidal resection. Out of the 17 women with infertility desiring pregnancy, 14 (82%) successfully conceived after surgery.[21]

CLINICAL OUTCOMES DURING PREGNANCY
Tumor Growth

During normal pregnancy, placental production of estrogen induces lactotroph hyperplasia with progressive increase in serum prolactin concentrations (up to 10 times the prepregnancy concentration in the third trimester) and enlargement of the normal pituitary gland.[22–24] In the healthy pregnant woman, pituitary volume increases by 45% in the first trimester and up to 136% by the end of pregnancy with return to prepregnancy size by 6 months postpartum.[25]

In women with prolactinomas, the stimulatory effects of estrogen can lead to tumor enlargement, which is often compounded by the discontinuation of DA therapy after pregnancy confirmation. In most cases, however, tumor enlargement is modest and not clinically significant. In a study of 100 women with prolactinomas, 37 underwent routine pituitary MRI scan without contrast injection between weeks 24 and 32 of gestation. After excluding 3 women who took DAs throughout pregnancy, tumor growth was observed in 66% of macroprolactinomas (8 out of 12, median increase of 3 mm) and 40% of microprolactinomas (9 out of 22, median increase of 0.5 mm). Only 14% (5 out of 34) were judged to have clinically significant tumor growth based on symptoms and/or optic chiasm contact.[26]

The risk of symptomatic tumor growth depends on prepregnancy tumor size and treatment. Molitch reviewed the published literature before 2015 and reported symptomatic tumor enlargement in 2.4% (18 out of 764) of microprolactinomas, 21.0% (50 out of 238) of macroprolactinomas treated only with DA,[27] and 4.7% (7 out of 148) of macroprolactinomas treated with prior surgery or radiation.[27] More recent studies, however, suggest higher rates of symptomatic tumor growth in macroprolactinomas treated with prior surgery (up to 33%), which may reflect different study populations and/or change in practice patterns.[28]

The duration of DA treatment before pregnancy may also affect outcomes. In a study of 22 patients with bromocriptine-induced pregnancies, Holgrem and colleagues found that at least 12 months of bromocriptine before pregnancy was protective against tumor growth.[29] In a study of 233 cabergoline-induced pregnancies, patients who had clinically significant tumor growth had a shorter median duration of cabergoline therapy before pregnancy (12 months) compared to those who had no significant tumor growth (24 months).[28]

Apoplexy

Pituitary apoplexy is rare during pregnancy and is caused by rapid tumor growth leading to increased intracapsular pressure, decreased blood flow, and hemorrhage.

Contributing factors include physiologic lactotroph hyperplasia, pituitary gland hyperemia, and a prothrombotic state during pregnancy. Apoplexy is potentially life-threatening for the mother and the fetus and presents with sudden-onset severe headache that can be associated with vision loss, cranial nerve palsies, nausea/vomiting, and less frequently meningism. New hormone deficiencies (adrenocorticotropic hormone [ACTH], thyroid-stimulating hormone, and rarely vasopressin) and electrolyte abnormalities (hyponatremia attributed to either ACTH deficiency or syndrome of inappropriate antidiuretic hormone secretion [SIADH]) can occur.

In a recent review of published reports of apoplexy during pregnancy, 43 total cases of apoplexy were identified. Of those, 26 had prolactinomas and 15 were on DA preconception. Apoplexy typically occurred in the second or third trimester (average week of gestation 26.4) with only one reported case in the first trimester.[30] In a separate case series and literature review focused on prolactinomas, 25 cases of apoplexy during pregnancy were identified. Preconception tumor size was greater than 1 cm in 12 cases, 1 cm or less in 9 cases, and not reported in 4 cases. Half of the cases were treated with the resumption of DA therapy, while the other half required surgery, usually due to deteriorating mental status or visual deficits.[31] The pregnancy course was usually favorable with healthy babies born at term. However, there was one neonatal death after premature delivery of twins at 28 weeks in a woman with giant prolactinoma with apoplexy at 22 weeks.[32]

Effect of Dopamine Agonist Therapy on the Developing Fetus

DAs are classified as pregnancy category B drugs (no increased risk in animal studies, inadequate human studies) by the US Food and Drug Administration.

Bromocriptine is an ergot alkaloid derivative with selective agonist activity at D2 and partial antagonist activity at D1 dopamine receptors and has been demonstrated to cross the placenta in human studies.[33] Compared to cabergoline, bromocriptine has a shorter half-life (which may reduce fetal exposure) and more published data on safety outcomes during pregnancy.[17,34]

The collective experience to date suggests that short-term exposure to bromocriptine during early pregnancy (less than 6 weeks) is not associated with an increased risk of maternal or fetal outcomes. In their review of 6272 bromocriptine-induced pregnancies (including women with nontumoral hyperprolactinemia), Huang and Molitch reported compiled rates of spontaneous abortions (9.9%), pregnancy terminations (1.2%), ectopic pregnancies (0.5%), hydatidiform moles (0.2%), preterm deliveries (12.5%), and congenital malformations (1.8%) similar to rates expected in the general population.[35]

Long-term follow-up studies (up to 20 years) in more than 1000 children whose mothers were treated with bromocriptine during early pregnancy have reported rare cases of developmental abnormalities including one case of tuberous sclerosis, one of idiopathic hydrocephalus, and one of precocious puberty.[36–38] Studies of bromocriptine throughout pregnancy in over 100 women have reported one case of undescended testes and one case of talipes deformity.[39,40]

Cabergoline is an ergot alkaloid derivative with selective agonist activity at dopamine D2 receptors. While human studies are lacking, cabergoline has been reported to cross the placenta in animal studies.[27,41]

A review of 1061 cabergoline-induced pregnancies suggest that short-term use of cabergoline during early pregnancy is safe with compiled rates of spontaneous abortions (7.5%), pregnancy terminations (6.5%), ectopic pregnancies (0.3%), hydatidiform moles (0.1%), preterm deliveries (10.1%), and congenital malformations (2.4%) similar to what is expected in the general population.[35,38] Long-term follow-up studies (up to 19 years) in 369 children whose mothers were treated with cabergoline have reported rates of developmental abnormalities ranging from 0% to 7% with 4 cases of epilepsy, 3 cases of language delay, 2 cases of autism spectrum disorder, and 1 case of attention deficit disorder.[26,28,42]

Data on the use of cabergoline through pregnancy is limited (less than 50 cases). In a recent study of 233 women with prolactinomas, those who were maintained on cabergoline had higher rates of miscarriage compared those who stopped DAs after pregnancy confirmation (38% vs 7.5%). However, additional details about the pregnancies were not available.[28]

A French database study of 183 women who received at least one DA prescription (bromocriptine or cabergoline) during pregnancy reported higher rates of pregnancy loss (adjusted prevalence OR 3.7, 95% confidence interval [CI] 1.8–7.4) and preterm birth (adjusted prevalence OR 3.6; 95% CI 1.5–8.3) in women prescribed DAs compared to matched controls. No difference in outcomes was observed in patients who received bromocriptine versus cabergoline.[43] Thus, while most of the safety data are reassuring, DAs should be discontinued once pregnancy is confirmed unless there is a specific reason to continue (eg, high risk of symptomatic tumor enlargement).

Other DAs such as quinagolide, pergolide, and lisuride are rarely used and/or no longer available. Short-term use of quinagolide has been reported in 176 pregnancies with increased rates of spontaneous abortions and fetal malformations and is, therefore, not recommended for use in women who desire pregnancy.[18]

APPROACH TO PATIENT MANAGEMENT
Preconception

The goals of preconception care in women with prolactinomas include (1) normalization of serum prolactin concentration, (2) restoration of ovulatory cycles, and (3) reduction of tumor size for large macroprolactinomas and/or those that are close to the optic chiasm. The last goal is also important to reduce the risk of symptomatic tumor growth during pregnancy. Medical and surgical options for treatment should be discussed with each patient.

Medical treatment with DAs is the recommended first-line therapy for women who are seeking pregnancy.[2,44] For the choice of DA, bromocriptine has been preferred by many in the past due to its shorter half-life and larger safety database. However, cabergoline use has increased in recent years due to its efficacy at normalizing prolactin and reducing tumor size, tolerability, and growing pregnancy safety record. In women who are already well-controlled on cabergoline, a switch to bromocriptine may lead to hyperprolactinemia that can adversely affect fertility. Thus, the European Society of Endocrinology (ESE) clinical practice guidelines and the Pituitary Society international consensus statement (weak recommendation) advise to use cabergoline at the lowest effective dose until pregnancy is confirmed and then discontinue upon pregnancy.[2,44] In general, women are advised to use mechanical contraception and track their menses during the first few months of DA therapy. This allows for prompt diagnosis of pregnancy and earlier discontinuation of DAs at 3 to 4 weeks of gestation.

In women with hyperprolactinemia and ovulatory cycles, treatment with DAs to normalize prolactin levels should still be considered. Luteal phase insufficiency affecting fertility can be an early consequence of hyperprolactinemia that precedes anovulation.

Women with large and/or invasive macroprolactinomas should have confirmation of treatment response (including tumor shrinkage) before attempting to conceive because of the higher risk of clinically significant tumor enlargement during pregnancy.[2,44] During this time, mechanical contraception should be used. In women who cannot tolerate DAs or who have inadequate response to medical therapy, transsphenoidal surgery prior to conception can be considered. Patients who undergo surgery should be counseled on the potential risk of hypopituitarism, although low if performed by an experienced pituitary surgeon. Radiotherapy is not recommended given the delayed onset of action and risk of hypopituitarism.

During Pregnancy

Once pregnancy is confirmed, DAs should be discontinued in most cases to reduce fetal exposure to the drug.[2,44] However, continuation of DAs during pregnancy can be considered in select cases after discussion of the risk and benefits. Possible scenarios for DA continuation include women with macroprolactinomas that are large and/or close to the optic chiasm or women with history of symptomatic tumor growth during prior pregnancies with an unplanned pregnancy on DAs. Safety data on the use of DAs throughout pregnancy are more limited than during early pregnancy alone.

Serum prolactin levels are not helpful in assessing prolactinoma status during pregnancy and should not be monitored.[2,44] Serum prolactin may not rise above what is expected during normal pregnancy and is not a reliable marker of tumor size.[45]

Monitoring during pregnancy depends on the size and location of the prolactinoma. Women with intrasellar microprolactinomas are at low risk of symptomatic tumor enlargement and can be followed clinically every trimester (**Box 2**). Women with

---

Box 2
Preconception, pregnancy, and postpartum care for women with prolactinomas

	Microprolactinomas	Macroprolactinomas (Especially if Abutting the Optic Chiasm)
Preconception	Discuss fertility potential, timeline for pregnancy, and pregnancy outcomes	
	In women desiring fertility, aim for normoprolactinemia and restoring ovulatory cycles	
	Use DAs at the lowest effective dose. Cabergoline is preferred given efficacy, tolerability, and safety profile.	
	Consider transsphenoidal surgery for DA resistance or intolerance	
	Advise that pregnancy can proceed without confirmation of tumor reduction	Delay pregnancy until treatment response is confirmed
Pregnancy confirmation	Discontinue DAs	May continue DAs in some cases (individualized recommendation)
During pregnancy	Perform a clinical evaluation each trimester	Perform a clinical evaluation monthly Obtain visual field examination each trimester
	Do not monitor prolactin levels	
	Repeat pituitary MRI without contrast and neuro-ophthalmology examination if mass effect symptoms develop	
	In patients with symptomatic tumor growth: restart DAs, consider surgery (in second trimester), and/or delivery (in third trimester)	
Postpartum	Advise that breastfeeding is not contraindicated unless DAs are required for tumor growth	
	Reassess prolactinoma status: clinical evaluation, prolactin measurement, and pituitary MRI	

Abbreviation: DA, dopamine agonist.

macroprolactinomas, especially those that are close to the optic chiasm, are at higher risk of symptomatic tumor enlargement and/or apoplexy and should undergo clinical evaluation every month and visual field examinations every trimester.[2,44]

If symptoms arise during pregnancy that are concerning for tumor enlargement (persistent/progressive headaches and visual field changes) or apoplexy (severe headaches, cranial nerve II, III, IV or VI palsy, and nausea/vomiting), a pituitary MRI without contrast should be obtained. MRI examinations are considered safe in pregnancy; however, gadolinium can cross the placenta and should not be utilized.[46–48]

In patients with demonstrated symptomatic tumor enlargement, treatment depends on the severity of symptoms and MRI findings. Options include (1) close monitoring, (2) reinitiation of DA therapy, (3) transsphenoidal surgery for tumor decompression, or (4) delivery if patient is close to her due date. Management should be individuated and discussed among a multidisciplinary team involving endocrinologists, neurosurgeons, neuro-ophthalmologists, and maternal–fetal care specialists.

Reinitiation of DAs has been demonstrated to be effective at relieving symptoms and reducing tumor size during pregnancy.[26] In our practice, we typically restart the DA that was effective for the patient preconception at doses similar or lower than the preconception dose.

Tumor decompression may be considered in select cases when patients do not respond to DA reinitiation and/or those with pituitary apoplexy with rapidly progressive visual symptoms or cranial nerve palsies and should be performed during the second trimester of pregnancy, if feasible.[2,44] For women in the third trimester of pregnancy, early delivery of the baby may be considered instead of transsphenoidal surgery.

Patients with tumor enlargement should also undergo the assessment for hypopituitarism. In particular, prompt glucocorticoid replacement and supportive treatment (eg, hemodynamic and electrolyte normalization) can be critical in patients with pituitary apoplexy.[49]

Postpartum

Breastfeeding

Breastfeeding is not contraindicated in most women postpartum and has not been associated with increased prolactin levels and/or symptoms of tumor enlargement.[50] However, DAs decrease breast milk production and should not be used during breastfeeding. Thus, breastfeeding is not advised in women with large macroprolactinomas that require ongoing medical treatment (eg, women reinitiated on DA therapy during pregnancy due to symptomatic tumor growth).

Reassessment of prolactinoma status

After pregnancy and lactation, women should undergo the reassessment of prolactinoma status. The ESE clinical practice guidelines recommend clinical evaluation, prolactin measurement, and MRI in case of previous macroprolactinoma 1 to 3 months after completion of breastfeeding.[44] Spontaneous remission of prolactinomas can occur after pregnancy due to autoinfarction of the tumor from hemodynamic changes during delivery and ranges from 10% to 68% (average 27.8%) in various studies.[51] Predictors of remission include older maternal age, smaller tumor size, and lower prolactin levels at the time of diagnosis as well as postpartum.[52–54]

In women who achieve remission after pregnancy and lactation, long-term monitoring is still warranted given the potential risk of recurrence. Late recurrences of prolactinomas have been described in up to 65% of women following cabergoline withdrawal[55] and is higher in those with remnant tumor on imaging despite biochemical remission.[56] Thus, clinical and hormonal follow-up is recommended at least once yearly in women whose prolactinomas are in remission.

SUMMARY

Prolactinomas commonly affect reproductive aged women and can present challenges for fertility. Medical treatment with DAs is effective at inducing pregnancy and can be stopped after pregnancy is detected in most women. Women with microprolactinomas typically have uneventful pregnancies with low risk of tumor enlargement. Women with large and/or invasive macroprolactinomas benefit from documented tumor reduction with DAs and/or surgery prior to conception. Rare cases of symptomatic tumor enlargement can occur during pregnancy and require close monitoring by a multidisciplinary team. Postpartum, breastfeeding is typically feasible, and all women should undergo evaluation for potential pregnancy-induced remission.

CLINICS CARE POINTS

- Aim for normoprolactinemia and restoration of ovulatory cycles in women with hyperprolactinemia who desire fertility.
- Discontinue dopamine agonist (DA) once pregnancy is confirmed.
- Assess for clinical symptoms of tumor enlargement and obtain a visual field exam each trimester in women with macroprolactinomas or microprolactinomas that abut the optic chiasm. Do not monitor prolactin levels during pregnancy.
- If symptomatic tumor enlargement occurs during pregnancy, consider restarting DA therapy, transsphenoidal surgery, or early delivery if near the due date.
- Re-evaluate prolactinoma status after pregnancy and advise patients that breast feeding is usually feasible in the absence of tumor growth.

DISCLOSURES

The authors have nothing to disclose.

REFERENCES

1. Chanson P, Maiter D. The epidemiology, diagnosis and treatment of Prolactinomas: The old and the new. Best Pract Res Clin Endocrinol Metabol 2019;33(2): 101290.
2. Petersenn S, Fleseriu M, Casanueva FF, et al. Diagnosis and management of prolactin-secreting pituitary adenomas: a Pituitary Society international Consensus Statement. Nat Rev Endocrinol 2023;19(12):722–40.
3. Lamba N, Noormohamed N, Simjian T, et al. Fertility after transsphenoidal surgery in patients with prolactinomas: A meta-analysis. Clin Neurol Neurosurg 2019;176:53–60.
4. Wong A, Eloy JA, Couldwell WT, et al. Update on prolactinomas. Part 1: Clinical manifestations and diagnostic challenges. J Clin Neurosci 2015;22(10):1562–7.
5. Knoppers BM, LeBris S. Recent advances in medically assisted conception: legal, ethical and social issues. Am J Law Med 1991;17(4):329–61.
6. Souter I, Baltagi LM, Toth TL, et al. Prevalence of hyperprolactinemia and abnormal magnetic resonance imaging findings in a population with infertility. Fertil Steril 2010;94(3):1159–62.

7. Molitch ME, Reichlin S. Hyperprolactinemic disorders. Dis Mon 1982;28(9):1–58.
8. Soto-Pedre E, Newey PJ, Bevan JS, et al. The epidemiology of hyperprolactinaemia over 20 years in the Tayside region of Scotland: the Prolactin Epidemiology, Audit and Research Study (PROLEARS). Clin Endocrinol 2017;86(1):60–7.
9. Millar RP, Sonigo C, Anderson RA, et al. Hypothalamic-pituitary-ovarian axis reactivation by kisspeptin-10 in hyperprolactinemic women with chronic amenorrhea. Journal of the Endocrine Society 2017;1(11):1362–71.
10. Brown RS, Herbison AE, Grattan DR. Prolactin regulation of kisspeptin neurones in the mouse brain and its role in the lactation-induced suppression of kisspeptin expression. J Neuroendocrinol 2014;26(12):898–908.
11. Sonigo C, Bouilly J, Carré N, et al. Hyperprolactinemia-induced ovarian acyclicity is reversed by kisspeptin administration. J Clin Invest 2012;122(10):3791–5.
12. Glass MR, Shaw RW, Butt WR, et al. An abnormality of oestrogen feedback in amenorrhoea-galactorrhoea. Br Med J 1975;3(5978):274–5.
13. Dorrington J, Gore-Langton RE. Prolactin inhibits oestrogen synthesis in the ovary. Nature 1981;290(5807):600–2.
14. Demura R, Ono M, Demura H, et al. Prolactin directly inhibits basal as well as gonadotropin-stimulated secretion of progesterone and 17β-estradiol in the human ovary. J Clin Endocrinol Metabol 1982;54(6):1246–50.
15. Corenblum B, Pairaudeau N, Shewchuk AB. Prolactin hypersecretion and short luteal phase defects. Obstet Gynecol 1976;47(4):486–8.
16. Seppälä M, Ranta T, Hirvonen E. Hyperprolactinaemia and luteal insufficiency. Lancet 1976;1(7953):229–30.
17. Webster J, Piscitelli G, Polli A, et al. A Comparison of Cabergoline and Bromocriptine in the Treatment of Hyperprolactinemic Amenorrhea. N Engl J Med 1994;331(14):904–9.
18. Webster J. A comparative review of the tolerability profiles of dopamine agonists in the treatment of hyperprolactinaemia and inhibition of lactation. Drug Saf 1996;14(4):228–38.
19. Ono M, Miki N, Amano K, et al. Individualized High-Dose Cabergoline Therapy for Hyperprolactinemic Infertility in Women with Micro- and Macroprolactinomas. J Clin Endocrinol Metabol 2010;95(6):2672–9.
20. Zamanipoor NAH, Zandbergen IM, de Vries F, et al. Surgery as a Viable Alternative First-Line Treatment for Prolactinoma Patients. A Systematic Review and Meta-Analysis. J Clin Endocrinol Metabol 2019;105(3):e32–41.
21. Yan Z, Wang Y, Shou X, et al. Effect of transsphenoidal surgery and standard care on fertility related indicators of patients with prolactinomas during child-bearing period. Int J Clin Exp Med 2015;8(11):21557–64.
22. Rigg LA, Lein A, Yen SS. Pattern of increase in circulating prolactin levels during human gestation. Am J Obstet Gynecol 1977;129(4):454–6.
23. Schock H, Zeleniuch-Jacquotte A, Lundin E, et al. Hormone concentrations throughout uncomplicated pregnancies: a longitudinal study. BMC Pregnancy Childbirth 2016;16(1):146.
24. Elster AD, Sanders TG, Vines FS, et al. Size and shape of the pituitary gland during pregnancy and post partum: measurement with MR imaging. Radiology 1991;181(2):531–5.
25. Cocks Eschler D, Javanmard P, Cox K, et al. Prolactinoma through the female life cycle. Endocrine 2018;59(1):16–29.
26. Lebbe M, Hubinont C, Bernard P, et al. Outcome of 100 pregnancies initiated under treatment with cabergoline in hyperprolactinaemic women. Clin Endocrinol (Oxf) 2010;73(2):236–42.

27. Molitch ME. Endocrinology in pregnancy: management of the pregnant patient with a prolactinoma. Eur J Endocrinol 2015;172(5):R205–13.

28. Sant' Anna BG, Musolino NRC, Gadelha MR, et al. A Brazilian multicentre study evaluating pregnancies induced by cabergoline in patients harboring prolactinomas. Pituitary 2020;23(2):120–8.

29. Holmgren U, Bergstrand G, Hagenfeldt K, et al. Women with prolactinoma–effect of pregnancy and lactation on serum prolactin and on tumour growth. Eur J Endocrinol 1986;111(4):452–9.

30. Gheorghe AM, Trandafir AI, Stanciu M, et al. Challenges of Pituitary Apoplexy in Pregnancy. J Clin Med 2023;12(10).

31. Kuhn E, Weinreich AA, Biermasz NR, et al. Apoplexy of microprolactinomas during pregnancy: report of five cases and review of the literature. Eur J Endocrinol 2021;185(1):99–108.

32. Khaldi S, Saad G, Elfekih H, et al. Pituitary apoplexy of a giant prolactinoma during pregnancy. Gynecol Endocrinol 2021;37(9):863–6.

33. BIGAZZI M, RONGA R, LANCRANJAN I, et al. A Pregnancy in an Acromegalic Woman during Bromocriptine Treatment: Effects on Growth Hormone and Prolactin in the Maternal, Fetal, and Amniotic Compartments. J Clin Endocrinol Metabol 1979;48(1):9–12.

34. Wang AT, Mullan RJ, Lane MA, et al. Treatment of hyperprolactinemia: a systematic review and meta-analysis. Syst Rev 2012;1:33.

35. Huang W, Molitch ME. Pituitary Tumors in Pregnancy. Endocrinol Metab Clin N Am 2019;48(3):569–81.

36. Bronstein MD. Prolactinomas and Pregnancy. Pituitary 2005;8(1):31–8.

37. Raymond JP, Goldstein E, Konopka P, et al. Follow-up of children born of bromocriptine-treated mothers. Horm Res 1985;22(3):239–46.

38. Krupp P, Monka C. Bromocriptine in pregnancy: safety aspects. Klin Wochenschr 1987;65(17):823–7.

39. Konopka P, Raymond JP, Merceron RE, et al. Continuous administration of bromocriptine in the prevention of neurological complications in pregnant women with prolactinomas. Am J Obstet Gynecol 1983;146(8):935–8.

40. Araujo B, Belo S, Carvalho D. Pregnancy and tumor outcomes in women with prolactinoma. Exp Clin Endocrinol Diabetes 2017;125(10):642–8.

41. Beltrame D, Longo M, Mazué G. Reproductive toxicity of cabergoline in mice, rats, and rabbits. Reprod Toxicol 1996;10(6):471–83.

42. Stalldecker G, Mallea-Gil MS, Guitelman M, et al. Effects of cabergoline on pregnancy and embryo-fetal development: retrospective study on 103 pregnancies and a review of the literature. Pituitary 2010;13(4):345–50.

43. Hurault-Delarue C, Montastruc J-L, Beau A-B, et al. Pregnancy outcome in women exposed to dopamine agonists during pregnancy: a pharmacoepidemiology study in EFEMERIS database. Arch Gynecol Obstet 2014;290(2):263–70.

44. Luger A, Broersen LHA, Biermasz NR, et al. ESE Clinical Practice Guideline on functioning and nonfunctioning pituitary adenomas in pregnancy. Eur J Endocrinol 2021;185(3):G1–33.

45. DIVERS Jr WA, YEN SS. Prolactin-producing microadenomas in pregnancy. Obstet Gynecol 1983;62(4):425–9.

46. Patenaude Y, Pugash D, Lim K, et al, Society of Obstetricians and Gynaecologists of Canada. RETIRED: the use of magnetic resonance imaging in the obstetric patient. J Obstet Gynaecol Can 2014;36(4):349–55.

47. Webb JA, Thomsen HS, Morcos SK, et al. The use of iodinated and gadolinium contrast media during pregnancy and lactation. Eur Radiol 2005;15:1234–40.

48. Committee Opinion No. 723: Guidelines for Diagnostic Imaging During Pregnancy and Lactation. Obstet Gynecol 2017;130(4):e210–6.
49. Grand'Maison S, Weber F, Bédard MJ, et al. Pituitary apoplexy in pregnancy: A case series and literature review. Obstet Med 2015;8(4):177–83.
50. Ikegami H, Aono T, Koizumi K, et al. Relationship between the methods of treatment for prolactinomas and the puerperal lactation. Fertil Steril 1987;47(5):867–9.
51. Auriemma RS, Pirchio R, Pivonello C, et al. Approach to the Patient With Prolactinoma. J Clin Endocrinol Metabol 2023;108(9):2400–23.
52. Domingue ME, Devuyst F, Alexopoulou O, et al. Outcome of prolactinoma after pregnancy and lactation: a study on 73 patients. Clin Endocrinol 2014;80(5): 642–8.
53. O'Sullivan SM, Farrant MT, Ogilvie CM, et al. An observational study of pregnancy and post-partum outcomes in women with prolactinoma treated with dopamine agonists. Aust N Z J Obstet Gynaecol 2020;60(3):405–11.
54. Tanrikulu S, Yarman S. Outcomes of Patients with Macroprolactinoma Desiring Pregnancy: Follow-Up to 23 Years from a Single Center. Horm Metab Res 2021; 53(06):371–6.
55. Hu J, Zheng X, Zhang W, et al. Current drug withdrawal strategy in prolactinoma patients treated with cabergoline: a systematic review and meta-analysis. Pituitary 2015;18:745–51.
56. Kharlip J, Salvatori R, Yenokyan G, et al. Recurrence of hyperprolactinemia after withdrawal of long-term cabergoline therapy. J Clin Endocrinol Metabol 2009; 94(7):2428–36.

Conundrums of Diagnosis and Management of Cushing's Syndrome in Pregnancy

Monica Livia Gheorghiu, MD, PhD[a,b], Maria Fleseriu, MD[c,d,e,*]

KEYWORDS

- Hypercortisolism • Pregnancy • Cushing's syndrome (CS) • Cushing's disease (CD)
- Diagnosis • Management • Treatment • Complications

KEY POINTS

- Pregnancy in women with CS is rare; in two-thirds of cases adrenal tumors (mostly benign) are present and in one-third of cases due to CD.
- A CS diagnosis during pregnancy is challenging due to overlap of signs and symptoms of normal pregnancy.
- In healthy pregnant women both serum and urinary cortisol, can be high, notably in the second and third trimester; however, circadian rhythm is preserved.
- Surgery during the second trimester (either pituitary or adrenal) is the main therapeutic choice for women who are diagnosed with CS during pregnancy.
- Care management by a specialized multidisciplinary team is recommended. Treatment of CS in women desiring pregnancy requires individualized planning.

INTRODUCTION

Endogenous Cushing's syndrome (CS) is a rare disease, with an estimated global, general population incidence of approximately 2 to 4.5 per million per year.[1,2] Although most patients are female individuals, pregnancy in women with CS is rare (~270 cases to date), with a prevalence estimated at 1 to 2 cases per 100,000 births.[3–5] The inhibitory effect of chronic hypercortisolism upon gonadotropin-releasing hormone pulsatile secretion, and consequently on gonadotropins, in addition to ovarian

[a] Department of Clinical Endocrinology IV, Carol Davila University of Medicine and Pharmacy Bucharest, Romania; [b] CI Parhon National Institute of Endocrinology, 34-36 Aviatorilor Boulevard, Sector 1, 011863, Bucharest, Romania; [c] Department of Medicine, Division of Endocrinology, Diabetes and Clinical Nutrition, Oregon Health & Science University, Portland, Oregon, USA; [d] Department of Neurological Surgery, Oregon Health & Science University, Portland, OR, USA; [e] Pituitary Center, Oregon Health & Science University, Portland, OR, USA
* Corresponding author. Oregon Health & Science University, Mail Code: CH8N, 3303 South Bond Avenue, Portland, OR 97239.
E-mail address: fleseriu@ohsu.edu

Endocrinol Metab Clin N Am 53 (2024) 421–435
https://doi.org/10.1016/j.ecl.2024.05.007
0889-8529/24/© 2024 Elsevier Inc. All rights reserved, including those for text and data mining, AI training, and similar technologies.
endo.theclinics.com

detrimental effects, leads to hypogonadotropic hypogonadism, oligomenorrhea or amenorrhea, anovulation, and infertility in more than 50% of cases.[6]

With augmented use of fertilization *in vitro* techniques, pregnancies in women with pituitary disorders, including Cushing's disease (CD) that is in remission, have significantly increased.[7] Overall, a high recurrence risk throughout lifetime(s) leads to the possibility that additional active CS during pregnancy cases will also occur and more studies are needed to access outcomes in such patients.[5,8]

Active CS during pregnancy is frequently associated with complications for both the mother and fetus.[9-11] Diagnosis of *de novo* CS or CS recurrence is difficult during gestation, due to an overlap of physiologic clinical and hormonal changes with those in patients with CS.[2,4,7,12] When considering the most appropriate treatment plan, it is important to take into account any potential adverse effects on the fetus.

This review will focus on the diagnosis and treatment challenges of CS during pregnancy.

ETIOLOGY OF CUSHING'S SYNDROME DURING PREGNANCY

Outside pregnancy, the leading cause of CS is CD in 60% to 70% of patients, while adrenal causes occur only in 20% to 30% of cases.[1,2] However, the etiology prevalence is reversed in pregnancy, with an adrenal origin accounting for approximately 60% (mostly adrenal adenomas; 44%–50%) of cases, CD in 28% to 34%, and adrenal carcinomas in 9% to 12%, while bilateral nodular hyperplasia or ectopic CS case is rarely observed.[5,10,11]

The causes of this discrepancy are not fully understood. Although androgens increase more in CD than in CS and may further contribute to the observed reduced pregnancy rate,[13] it seems menstrual irregularities in women with CS are more correlated with hypercortisolism severity rather than with androgen levels.[14]

Interestingly, in 2 retrospective studies, more than a quarter (27%) of women of reproductive age with CD became symptomatic during gestation or over the 12 months following pregnancy (defined as pregnancy-associated CD).[15,16] The physiologic hyperactivity of the hypothalamic-pituitary-adrenal (HPA) axis during gestation was proposed as a mechanism for either corticotroph adenoma formation or activation during pregnancy and peripartum.[15] Corticotroph adenomas may express estrogen receptors; however, a direct proliferative effect of estrogens has not been described.[8] Furthermore, pregnancy seems to neither increase CD recurrence in women with CD cured after pituitary surgery[17] nor accelerate corticotroph tumor progression in patients after bilateral adrenalectomy (BLA), although plasma adrenocorticotropic hormone (ACTH) and pituitary adenoma volume may increase during pregnancy.[18]

Transient pregnancy-induced CS that usually subsides following delivery (but may recur in subsequent gestations) has been described in some cases of ACTH-independent CS. Aberrant adrenal gland receptors may lead to an increased cortisol production during pregnancy in response to human chorionic gonadotropin, luteinizing hormone-releasing hormone, glucagon, vasopressin, estradiol, or after a meal.[19,20] Interestingly, these receptors have been described in both apparently normal adrenal glands, as well as in adrenal adenomas, carcinomas, or bilateral nodular adrenal hyperplasia[21] and may account for the higher rate of adrenal CS in pregnancy.

COMPLICATIONS OF CUSHING'S SYNDROME IN PREGNANCY

Patients with CS have an increased risk of comorbidities and higher mortality mostly due to cardiovascular disorders.[2] Furthermore, CS during pregnancy can be associated with severe maternal and fetal complications; therefore, women with active CS should be counseled to avoid pregnancy.[5]

Several multicenter or systematic retrospective reviews on CS in pregnancy have been published, describing maternal and fetal complications and outcome with or without active treatment during pregnancy. For example, 3 large series with CS cases (mostly adrenal, but also CD) included 136 pregnancies,[11] 263 pregnancies,[10] and 135 pregnancies that were compared with greater than 9 million non-CS control pregnancies[3] (**Table 1**). Smaller more recent series have evaluated only CD cases, potentially with more severe CS than those of adrenal origin: 62 pregnancies (13 with transsphenoidal surgery [TSS] and 9 with medical treatment),[22] 21 pregnancies in women with active hypercortisolism compared to pregnancies with CD after TSS before pregnancy (25 eucortisolic and 32 with hypocortisolism on replacement) and with the general population[23] (see **Table 1**). Another retrospective surgical series observed 19 pregnancies in women with pregnancy-associated CD (developed clinically in the year following pregnancy in most of them) compared with 30 women with pregnancies greater than 12 months before CD.[16] However, different proportions of these patients have been diagnosed with CS during the first 12 months after pregnancy or may have been treated (either surgically or/and medically) during pregnancy.

Maternal complications are very frequent, occurring in 50% to 70% of patients. Examples include hypertension (40%–68%), preeclampsia (14%–26%), impaired glucose tolerance or diabetes mellitus (26%–37%), osteoporosis (5%), fractures, poor wound healing and infections (2%), severe psychiatric complications (4%), cardiac failure (2%), and even death (0.7%–2%)[3,5,9,11,13,22,23] (see **Table 1**). Women with CS are more likely to be older, obese, with chronic hypertension and pregestational diabetes during pregnancy versus control women without hypercortisolemia; adjusted odds ratio for preeclampsia is 2.2 ($P < .001$).[3]

Furthermore, women with active CS reportedly experienced significantly more complications than those experienced by women with cured CS, for example, diabetes mellitus (36.9% vs 2.3%), hypertension (40.5% vs 2.3%), and preeclampsia (26.3% vs 2.3%).[10] The cesarean rate was also higher (51.7% vs 21.9%).[10] Operative vaginal delivery and blood transfusion risks were increased in active CS compared to non-CS controls.[3] Maternal mortality in active CS is also increased, 1257 out of 100,000 population (6 fold higher than that worldwide, as reported in 2013).[10] In another study, maternal mortality rate was 0.7% in CS and 0.007% in the control group.[3]

Fetal complications are also numerous, for example, prematurity (33%–66%), early spontaneous abortion or intrauterine death (5%–31%), intrauterine growth restriction, low birth weight (21%–68%), respiratory distress, hypoglycemia, and hypoadrenalism.[10,11,23] The complication risk is increased in women with active CS during pregnancy, notably in those individuals diagnosed *de novo* during pregnancy[10,23] (see **Table 1**). Prematurity (birth <37 gestation weeks) is a more frequent occurrence in women with active hypercortisolism compared to those with cured CS and eucortisolism (33% vs 8%), being highest (62.5%) when CS was diagnosed during pregnancy.[23] Fetal loss and global fetal morbidity are also higher in women with active disease versus those with cured CS (23.6% vs 8.5% and 33.3% vs 4.9%, respectively).[10] However, CS during gestation was not associated with any specific malformations.[5,10,11,22,23]

Rates of maternal and fetal complications are reported as comparable in active CD[22,23] and CS cases series of different etiologies[3,10,11] (see **Table 1**). Risk tended to be higher in women with active hypercortisolism in pregnancy, when compared to treated patients, albeit with small groups and different severities of CD in treated and untreated patients. In CS in remission, both maternal and fetal risks tend to be

Table 1
The most frequent complications in pregnant women with Cushing's syndrome

Study Population	Lindsay et al,[11] 2005	Caimari et al,[10] 2017		Baghlaf et al,[3] 2022 (US Population)		Sridharan et al,[22] 2021	Hochman et al,[23] 2021 (French Population)	
	CS[a] (n = 136)	Active CS (n = 214)	Cured CS (n = 49)	CS (n = 135)	Non-CS (n = 9,096,653)	CD[a] (n = 62)	Active CD (n = 21)	Cured CD Eucortisolemic (n = 25)
Pregnant women								
Hypertension, %	68	40.5	2.3	16.3	7.4	19.1	19	4
Preeclampsia, %	14	26.3	2.3	8.1	3.6	21.2	9.5	0
Gestational diabetes mellitus, %	25[b]	36.9	2.3	8.1	5.8	21.2	47.6	12
Cesarean delivery, %	n/a	51.7	21.9	32.6	32.3	42.1	23.8	12
Assisted vaginal delivery, %	n/a	n/a	n/a	30.4	6.5	n/a	n/a	n/a
Fetus								
Prematurity, %	43	65.8	2.5	8.9	7.2	50.9	33[c]	8[c]
Fetal loss, %	11	23.6	8.5	n/a	n/a	13	4.8	0
Low birth weight/IUGR, %	21	71	16	n/a	n/a	59	n/a	n/a

Abbreviations: CS, Cushing's syndrome; CD, Cushing's disease; IUGR, intrauterine growth restriction.; n/a, not available.
[a] Overall cohort (treated and untreated patients).
[b] Included IGT (impaired glucose tolerance).
[c] (P = .059). Statistically significant higher prevalence of complications in patients with active disease versus control groups are shown in **bold** text.

similar with those in the general population.[10,23] Therefore, it is mandatory to establish early the diagnosis of CS, especially during pregnancy, to avoid the detrimental consequences of untreated hypercortisolism.

DIAGNOSIS OF CUSHING'S SYNDROME DURING PREGNANCY
Clinical Picture

There is a considerable overlap between many CS signs and symptoms and those signs and symptoms that may occur in normal pregnancies, for example, preeclampsia, gestational diabetes mellitus or pregnancy-associated weight gain, abdominal pink striae, hypertension, fatigue, hyperglycemia, and mood changes.

More specific signs for CS are easy bruising, myopathy, wide, violaceous striae (in particular, when they are large and/or located outside abdominal area), pathologic fractures, difficult to control hypertension, and hyperglycemia.[9,24] A history of previous hypertension, type 2 diabetes mellitus, preeclampsia, or fetal loss may be encountered in patients with CS.[25] In cases of suggestive clinical features, a detailed anamnesis should exclude iatrogenic sources of glucocorticoids,[1] with oral, injectable, topical, inhalation, or intranasal administration.[24]

Most importantly, in pregnancy, only those women with strongly suggestive clinical features for CS should undergo laboratory testing.[5]

Laboratory Diagnosis

A hormonal workup during pregnancy should evaluate the following:

- Disease severity in a pregnant woman with known CS (more likely with persistent CD),
- CD recurrence in a previously treated woman with CD, and
- *de novo* CS during pregnancy (or reject the suspicion in a pregnant woman with more severe clinical signs, hypertension, diabetes mellitus, or glucose intolerance).

Diagnostic pitfalls may be due to the physiologic changes in the HPA axis during normal pregnancy.

MATERNAL AND FETAL CHANGES IN THE HYPOTHALAMIC-PITUITARY-ADRENAL AXIS IN PREGNANCY

Normal human pregnancy is accompanied by a significant increase in maternal HPA axis activity, leading to a state of physiologic hypercortisolism. There is a rise in corticotropin-releasing hormone (CRH), ACTH, and free and total cortisol levels, but with diurnal cortisol biorhythm maintenance.[12,26]

The placenta secretes, in a noncircadian manner, placental CRH (pCRH) starting from the first trimester, with a marked increase during the second and third trimesters and a peak before labor. Having a similar structure with maternal CRH, pCRH stimulates ACTH secretion, which in turn stimulates adrenal cortisol production. ACTH (from maternal and placental sources) increases progressively during pregnancy (but not proportionally with CRH levels) and peaks during labor (up to 10 fold in the nonpregnant range). These prelabor changes may contribute to the initiation of parturition (CRH), to maternal preparation for the stress of labor, and to the final stages of fetal organ development before birth.[12,26–28]

Elevated placental estrogens increase corticosteroid-binding globulin (CBG) hepatic production, which contributes to a gradual increase in total cortisol levels (from 1.6 fold by the end of the first trimester to 2.4 fold in the second trimester and up to

3 fold nonpregnant levels in the third trimester).[29,30] Rising progesterone levels induce cortisol resistance and cortisol displacement from CBG, contributing to a further increase in free cortisol levels[26] (**Fig. 1**).

Free cortisol and, in particular, urinary free cortisol (UFC) levels are elevated in normal pregnancies, with UFC rising to 1.8 to 2 fold nonpregnant levels during the second trimester and up to a 3 fold increase in the third trimester.[5,28–30]

Late-night salivary cortisol rises progressively during normal pregnancies, with up to a 2 fold increase in the third trimester. The cortisol circadian biorhythm is still maintained, but with a reduced level of fluctuation occurring, notably during the third trimester.[31,32]

There is also a decreased sensitivity of the pituitary corticotrophs to cortisol's negative feedback inhibition. Together with the increased levels of total serum cortisol, these may explain the reduced cortisol inhibition occurring after an overnight dexamethasone suppression test.[33]

In late pregnancy, increased cortisol levels downregulate maternal CRH production, leading to corticotroph cells desensitization, which may also explain an attenuated response to exogenous CRH.[26]

The fetus is partially protected from maternal hypercortisolism by placental 11-β-hydroxysteroid dehydrogenase 2 (11beta-HSD2), located mostly on the fetal side of the fetoplacental unit. The enzyme inactivates cortisol by conversion to cortisone, metabolizing 80% to 90% of maternal circulating cortisol. Despite this, 25% of fetal cortisol at term is derived from the mother, and excessive maternal glucocorticoids may overwhelm placental 11beta-HSD2, with detrimental effects for the fetus.[28,34]

After delivery, CRH and ACTH levels rapidly decrease, with ACTH normalization 24 hours after delivery. Maternal serum and salivary cortisol, as well as free cortisol levels, are likely to return to baseline after 1 week, but the restoration timeline may vary. CBG levels return to prepregnant levels with variable time frames, occurring from 3 weeks to 3 months postdelivery. Normal cortisol suppression post-dexamethasone may take up to 5 weeks after birth, and by 2 to 3 months, cortisol and UFC levels have typically normalized.[5,35,36]

PRACTICAL TIPS FOR DIAGNOSIS OF CUSHING'S SYNDROME DURING PREGNANCY
Biochemical Workup

Screening

- *24 hour UFC level* above normal in the first trimester, greater than 3 fold nonpregnant values in the second and third trimesters are suggestive for CS (increases up to 2–3 fold are not discriminative during this period). Repeat at least 2 to 4 UFC specimens.[5,25]
- *Late-night salivary cortisol* levels greater than 2 fold nonpregnant values (second and third trimesters), with blunted circadian rhythm, are highly suggestive for CS; proposed cutoff values for cortisol enzyme-linked immunosorbent assay (Salimetrics, LLC, Carlsbad, CA) kit: 7.0, 7.2, and 7.9 nmol/L for first, second, and third trimesters, respectively—sensitivity of 80% to 92% and specificity of 93% to 100% in the diagnosis of CD.[32] Establishing cutoffs for other assays is required.
- *Morning total cortisol* levels less than 2 to 3 fold nonpregnant values are not suggestive for a diagnosis.
- *Overnight or low-dose dexamethasone suppression tests* (2 mg/d for 2 days) are not reliable and not recommended during pregnancy (insufficient cortisol

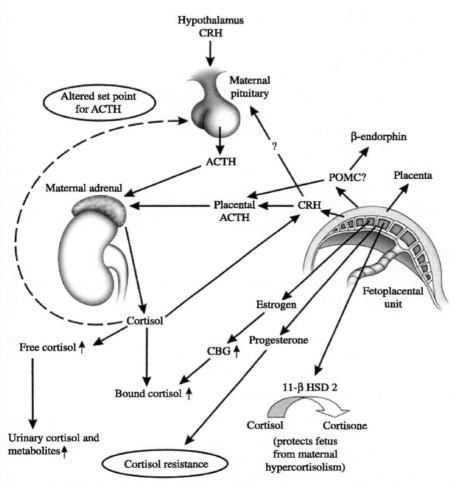

Fig. 1. Role of the fetoplacental unit in HPA axis changes in pregnancy.[28] Maternal total and free cortisol increase during pregnancy. Elevated estrogen levels stimulate hepatic production of CBG, resulting in total serum cortisol elevation. Total and free cortisol levels also increase in response to placental corticotropin-releasing hormone and placental ACTH that rise progressively throughout pregnancy. pCRH is under positive feedback control by cortisol, but its effect on the maternal pituitary is unclear. Pregnancy is also a state of adrenal hyperresponsivity to ACTH. The HPA axis appears to be reset at a higher level in pregnancy due to cortisol resistance induced by rising progesterone levels. Progesterone also displaces cortisol from CBG, further elevating free cortisol levels. The fetus is protected from maternal hypercortisolism by inactivation to cortisone by placental 11-β-hydroxysteroid dehydrogenase 2. POMC, proopiomelanocortin; CBG, corticosteroid-binding globulin; 11β-HSD 2, 11β-hydroxysteroid dehydrogenase 2; ACTH, adrenocorticotropic hormone; pCRH, placental corticotropin-releasing hormone. (Z Karaca, F Tanriverdi, K Unluhizarci, F Kelestimur, Pregnancy and pituitary disorders, European Journal of Endocrinology, Volume 162, Issue 3, Mar 2010, Pages 453–475, https://doi.org/10.1530/EJE-09-0923.)

suppression, high false-positive rates in up to 60% at 1 mg overnight test).[5,11,33]

Biochemical Localization Testing

- *Morning ACTH* levels in CD may be in the higher normal range or above; in CS from adrenal causes, while ACTH may not be suppressed, ACTH is actually in the lower part of the nonpregnant range in about 50% of CS cases.[5,11]
- *High-dose dexamethasone suppression test* (8 mg/d for 2 days) is not recommended in pregnancy, as there is insufficient experience/evidence; a greater than 80% fall in cortisol has been reported to distinguish between adrenal and pituitary source of CS in pregnancy.[5,11]
- *Desmopressin or CRH stimulation* test for CD diagnosis: limited experience, CRH not available; not recommended in pregnancy; and cortisol stimulation (absent in healthy pregnant women) was present in a few reported cases.[11,37]
- *Bilateral inferior petrosal sinus sampling* is usually not recommended during pregnancy due to the risk of radiation and venous thromboembolism.[5]

Imaging

- *Pituitary MRI:* Is needed when CD is suspected, but greater than 40% of microadenomas may not be visible. Notably, there is a physiologic increase in pituitary volume during pregnancy. Although gadolinium use has not been associated with fetal anomalies, MRI should be performed preferably without gadolinium (in particular, during the first trimester).[5,26]
- *Adrenal imaging:* Adrenal ultrasound (preferably) or abdominal MRI without contrast may identify an adrenal cause. Computed tomography is not recommended during pregnancy due to radiation risk.

MANAGEMENT OF CUSHING'S SYNDROME DURING PREGNANCY

Treatment of CS in women desiring pregnancy requires individualized planning, especially in CD cases, where the recurrence rate post-TSS is high.[4] Repeat pituitary surgery for women with active CD, as well as radiation carry a higher risk of hypopituitarism, which could impact fertility. Medical treatment is not approved for use in pregnancy. Thus, BLA is frequently recommended for patients desiring pregnancy.[4,25]

Pregnant women with CS should be managed by a highly specialized multidisciplinary team.[4] A team with experience in pituitary and high-risk pregnancies, a team equipped with the experience needed to address systemic maternal complications and to monitor fetal evolution and manage potential complicated deliveries as well as neonatal morbidity.

Due to limited experience (less than 100 cases treated surgically or medically during pregnancy), increased mother and fetus risks with active disease, lack of any drug approved for CS treatment during pregnancy, and potential benefits and risks of pituitary or adrenal surgery, the approach should be individualized and patients well informed about all the therapeutic options.[38,39] Pituitary radiotherapy is not recommended for CD in pregnancy, due to the risk of fetal birth defects.

CONSERVATIVE MANAGEMENT (OBSERVATION)

In patients with mild hypercortisolism, notably if diagnosed in late pregnancy, close observation with optimal treatment of mother's comorbidities (hypertension and diabetes) and regular monitoring may be an option.[2,4,5,38]

MANAGEMENT OF COMPLICATIONS

Thromboprophylaxis with low molecular weight heparin should be strongly considered given the increased risk for venous thrombotic events (VTEs) both in pregnancy and in CD. Odds ratio of spontaneous VTEs in CS is 18% versus non-CS population,[40] and antithrombotic prophylaxis can reduce morbidity and mortality. Special consideration is needed perioperatively for all patients with CS, but, especially for pregnant women.[5,25] Other complications, when present should also be addressed in parallel with CS treatment, including diabetes mellitus, hypertension, and cardiovascular disorders.

SURGERY

In women who develop severe CD while pregnant, the main treatment option is surgery (pituitary adenomectomy or laparoscopic adrenalectomy, either unilateral for adrenal tumors or bilateral for refractory CD, bilateral nodular hyperplasia, or rare ectopic ACTH secretion).[4,5,39] The second trimester, when fetal loss or preterm birth risk is lower, is a preferred time for surgical intervention.[5,39]

However, surgical outcome data are scarce. In one study, 13 women with CD underwent TSS at a mean gestational age of 17 ± 3.7 weeks with a remission rate of 77%.[22] In a systematic review[10] reporting outcomes on a total of 61 women who had undergone surgery, 11 had TSS, 44 unilateral adrenalectomies, and 6 bilateral adrenalectomies during pregnancy. Fetal loss rate was significantly lower if women were in remission postsurgery versus those not in remission (6.7% vs 28.6%), while preterm birth (56.1% vs 80%), and low birth weight rate also tended to decrease (70.6% vs 100%).[10] A laparoscopic approach was reportedly well tolerated.[41]

In cases of adrenocortical carcinoma, some experts suggest that unilateral adrenalectomy may be undertaken in any trimester, but the prognosis for both mother and fetus is generally poor.[39]

Adrenal insufficiency either after adrenalectomy or after pituitary surgery is very common and should be actively tested for and treated with physiologic replacement doses of hydrocortisone. Dexamethasone should not be used in pregnancy.[28,42] Hydrocortisone doses may be increased by 20% to 40% in the second or third trimester, if clinically required, to ensure adequate replacement.[28,42] In a French multicenter retrospective study of women with previous or current CS at the time of pregnancy,[23] the premature birth rate was 33% in women with hypercortisolism, 19.3% in those with hypocortisolism after previous CS treatment (despite apparently adequate hydrocortisone replacement during pregnancy, 22–24 mg/d), and only 8% in women with cured CS and eucortisolism during pregnancy (comparable to the rate in the normal population).[23]

MEDICAL TREATMENT

Although no drugs are approved for CS treatment during pregnancy, medical treatment may be rarely considered for patients with active, severe, complicated CS diagnosed during pregnancy (in the first and third trimesters in particular) and in those who are waiting on surgery or pose considerable maternal or fetal risks[5,38,39] (**Table 2**).

In women with CD and chronic medical treatment after unsuccessful pituitary surgery, the benefits and potential risks of medical treatment during pregnancy should be thoroughly discussed. Experts recommend considering BLA for women with non-cured CD who plan for pregnancy.[4,5]

Table 2
Medical therapy used in pregnant women with active Cushing's syndrome. All medications are used off-label for Cushing's syndrome

Drug(ref)	No of Pregnancies (n = 40)	Doses Used in Pregnancy	Side Effects/Risks	Observations
Metyrapone[10,11,13,39,44-49]	22 (4 CD)	500–3000 mg/d in 2–3 doses	• Hypertension aggravation • Preeclampsia • Hypokalemia • Increased maternal androgens • Risk of adrenal insufficiency in mother and neonate	• Drug with largest experience in pregnancy • Mostly initiated in trimester 2 or 3 • Generally well tolerated • Crosses the placenta, it is excreted in breast milk • Pregnancy risk class C • Scarce experience with breastfeeding
Ketoconazole[11,13,39,49-52]	7 (3 CD)	400–1000 mg/d in 2–4 doses	• Increased liver enzymes • Adrenal insufficiency • Risk of feminization of male fetus if given during first trimester (not observed in 1 case[50])	• Teratogenic and risk for abortion in animal studies (not seen in reported human cases, in 3 used during first trimester) • Pregnancy risk class C • Not recommended during breastfeeding
Cabergoline[52,54-57]	5 (all CD, monotherapy in 4 cases)	0.5–2 mg/wk (1 case 10 mg/wk)	• Impairs postpartum lactation • Generally well tolerated	• Use restricted to CD • Mild efficacy • Overall safe for fetus (large experience in prolactinomas) • Pregnancy risk class B
Cyproheptadine[11,38]	3 (all CD)		• Somnolence • Increased appetite	• Not used anymore for CS due to low efficacy rate
Aminoglutethimide[11]	1 (CD)		• Risk of masculinization in female fetus	• Not recommended
Mitotane[5,38]	2 (CD)		• Teratogenic	• Not recommended during pregnancy

Abbreviations: CD, Cushing's disease; CS, Cushing's syndrome.

Considering the physiologically elevated UFC level in normal pregnancy, the recommended target for medical treatment is a 1.5 fold UFC level compared to normal nonpregnant reference ranges.[25]

Metyrapone, an 11-ß hydroxylase inhibitor, has a quick action onset.[4,25,43] Close surveillance is required for worsening hypertension, preeclampsia, hypokalemia (due to mineralocorticoid precursors increasing), increased androgens, and risk of adrenal insufficiency.[5,38] Although no fetal congenital defects have been reported to date,[10,11,13,39,44–49] metyrapone crosses the placental barrier[44] leading to a potential risk of fetal adrenal insufficiency or changes in adrenal steroidogenesis. Long-term metyrapone effects in pregnancy are unknown.[5]

Ketoconazole inhibits multiple enzymes involved in adrenal steroidogenesis.[4,25,43] Although in animal studies ketoconazole is teratogenic and associated with an increased risk of abortion, in humans, these risks were not reported.[11,13,39,49–52] Side effects include gastrointestinal disturbances, increased liver enzymes, skin rash, adrenal insufficiency, and risk of feminization in male fetus if given during the first trimester (not confirmed in 1 reported case[50]).

Cabergoline is a dopamine agonist important for treatment during pregnancy in selected women with prolactinomas.[53] Used off-label in CD treatment,[4,25,43] overall, cabergoline was well tolerated in the few reported cases, in doses of 0.5 to 3.5 mg (and up to 10 mg) per week in pregnancy.[52,54–57] Potential side effects are impaired lactation, headache, nasal congestion, hypotension, depression, dizziness, and increased impulse control disorders.

Treatment of CS during pregnancy was associated with a decreased rate of fetal loss in a retrospective systematic review; 20.8% in medically treated women, 12.5% in surgically treated mothers compared to 30.6% in nontreated mothers ($P < .05$).[10] However, prematurity, intrauterine growth restriction, and low birth weight risks did not decrease significantly in those treated medically or surgically during pregnancy.[10]

To date, there are no reported cases of CS treatment during pregnancy with other drugs approved for CS, for example, pasireotide, osilodrostat, or levoketoconazole.

DRUGS NOT TO BE USED IN CUSHING'S SYNDROME DURING PREGNANCY

Mitotane (an adrenolytic drug used for advanced adrenocortical carcinoma)—potential teratogenic effect.[5]

Mifepristone (nonselective glucocorticoid receptor antagonist)—risk of abortion.

SUMMARY

Pregnancy is rare in women with CS, but active CS poses many risks for both mother and fetus, and women should be managed by an expert multidisciplinary team. A diagnosis is challenging due to the overlap with clinical and biochemical changes that occur in normal pregnancies. All biochemical tests have potential pitfalls and furthermore, normal ranges differ from those outside pregnancy. The first line of treatment is surgery (preferably in the second trimester). In severe cases, medical therapy, for example, metyrapone, or cabergoline might be rarely considered, although these medical therapies are not approved for use in pregnancy. Remission after treatment improves the risk of fetal loss, but other fetal complications (prematurity and low birth weight) may remain increased. In patients with CD in remission before pregnancy, especially if they are eucortisolemic, there seems to be no significant increased risk compared to the general population. However, the risk of CD recurrence is high, and patients need close follow-up and testing during pregnancy if there is a clinical suspicion of recurrence.

CLINICS CARE POINTS

- Most women with CS diagnosed during pregnancy have adrenal CS.
- As both urine and serum cortisol are high in normal pregnancy, salivary cortisol is the preferred diagnostic tests for CS in pregnancy.
- Surgery is the first-line treatment of most patients with pituitary and adrenal adenomas diagnosed in pregnancy. Surgery is recommended to be performed in the second trimester for best outcomes for both mother and baby.
- In selected cases with very mild disease, especially in the third trimester, observation has also been suggested.
- There are no medications approved for CS treatment in pregnancy; however, a few drugs have been used with various success. A target posttreatment is a 1.5 fold UFC level.
- Anticoagulation (mostly low molecular weight heparin) should be carefully considered as CS increases the risk of thromboembolism, which is already increased in pregnancy.
- Management by a specialized multidisciplinary team is recommended.
- Due to an elevated risk of complications, women with active CS should be counseled not to get pregnant before achieving disease remission.
- Treatment of CS in women desiring pregnancy requires individualized planning; BLA is preferred for women in these cases.

DISCLOSURE

M. L. Gheorghiu reports no potential conflict of interest relevant to this article. M. Fleseriu has received research support to Oregon Health & Science University as a principal investigator from Recordati, Sparrow, and Xeris and has served as occasional scientific consultant to Recordati, Sparrow, and Xeris.

REFERENCES

1. Gadelha M, Gatto F, Wildemberg LE, et al. Cushing's syndrome. Lancet 2023; 402:2237–52.
2. Reincke M, Fleseriu M. Cushing Syndrome: A Review. JAMA 2023;330:170–81.
3. Baghlaf HA, Badeghiesh AM, Suarthana E, et al. The effect of Cushing's syndrome on pregnancy complication rates: analysis of more than 9 million deliveries. J Matern Fetal Neonatal Med 2022;35:6236–42.
4. Fleseriu M, Varlamov EV, Hinojosa-Amaya JM, et al. An individualized approach to the management of Cushing disease. Nat Rev Endocrinol 2023;19:581–99.
5. Luger A, Broersen LHA, Biermasz NR, et al. ESE Clinical Practice Guideline on functioning and nonfunctioning pituitary adenomas in pregnancy. Eur J Endocrinol 2021;185:G1–33.
6. Castinetti F, Brue T. Impact of Cushing's syndrome on fertility and pregnancy. Ann Endocrinol 2022;83:188–90.
7. Vila G, Fleseriu M. Fertility and pregnancy in women with hypopituitarism: a systematic literature review. J Clin Endocrinol Metab 2020;105:dgz112.
8. Melmed S, Kaiser UB, Lopes MB, et al. Clinical biology of the pituitary adenoma. Endocr Rev 2022;43:1003–37.

9. Bronstein MD, Machado MC, Fragoso MC. Management of endocrine disease: Management of pregnant patients with Cushing's syndrome. Eur J Endocrinol 2015;173:R85–91.
10. Caimari F, Valassi E, Garbayo P, et al. Cushing's syndrome and pregnancy outcomes: a systematic review of published cases. Endocrine 2017;55:555–63.
11. Lindsay JR, Jonklaas J, Oldfield EH, et al. Cushing's syndrome during pregnancy: personal experience and review of the literature. J Clin Endocrinol Metab 2005;90:3077–83.
12. Lindsay JR, Nieman LK. The hypothalamic-pituitary-adrenal axis in pregnancy: challenges in disease detection and treatment. Endocr Rev 2005;26:775–99.
13. Machado MC, Fragoso MCBV, Bronstein MD. Pregnancy in patients with Cushing's Syndrome. Endocrinol Metab Clin North Am 2018;47:441–9.
14. Lado-Abeal J, Rodriguez-Arnao J, Newell-Price JD, et al. Menstrual abnormalities in women with Cushing's disease are correlated with hypercortisolemia rather than raised circulating androgen levels. J Clin Endocrinol Metab 1998;83:3083–8.
15. Palejwala SK, Conger AR, Eisenberg AA, et al. Pregnancy-associated Cushing's disease? An exploratory retrospective study. Pituitary 2018;21:584–92.
16. Tang K, Lu L, Feng M, et al. The incidence of pregnancy-associated Cushing's Disease and its relation to pregnancy: a retrospective study. Front Endocrinol 2020;11:305.
17. Lousada LM, Tapia MJB, Cescato VAS, et al. Pregnancy after pituitary surgery does not influence the recurrence of Cushing's disease. Endocrine 2022;78:552–8.
18. Jornayvaz FR, Assie G, Bienvenu-Perrard M, et al. Pregnancy does not accelerate corticotroph tumor progression in Nelson's syndrome. J Clin Endocrinol Metab 2011;96:E658–62.
19. Caticha O, Odell WD, Wilson DE, et al. Estradiol stimulates cortisol production by adrenal cells in estrogen-dependent primary adrenocortical nodular dysplasia. J Clin Endocrinol Metab 1993;77:494–7.
20. Li Y, Lin J, Fu S, et al. The mystery of transient pregnancy-induced cushing's syndrome: a case report and literature review highlighting GNAS somatic mutations and LHCGR overexpression. Endocrine 2024;83:473–82.
21. El Gorayeb N, Bourdeau I, Lacroix A. Multiple aberrant hormone receptors in Cushing's syndrome. Eur J Endocrinol 2015;173:M45–60.
22. Sridharan K, Sahoo J, Palui R, et al. Diagnosis and treatment outcomes of Cushing's disease during pregnancy. Pituitary 2021;24:670–80.
23. Hochman C, Cristante J, Geslot A, et al. Pre-term birth in women exposed to Cushing's disease: the baby-cush study. Eur J Endocrinol 2021;184:469–76.
24. Scutelnicu A, Panaitescu AM, Ciobanu AM, et al. Iatrogenic Cushing's syndrome as a consequence of nasal use of Betamethasone spray during pregnancy. Acta Endocrinol 2020;16:511–7.
25. Fleseriu M, Auchus R, Bancos I, et al. Consensus on diagnosis and management of Cushing's disease: a guideline update. Lancet Diabetes Endocrinol 2021;9:847–75.
26. Karaca Z, Tanriverdi F, Unluhizarci K, et al. Pregnancy and pituitary disorders. Eur J Endocrinol 2010;162:453–75.
27. Thomson M. The physiological roles of placental corticotropin releasing hormone in pregnancy and childbirth. J Physiol Biochem 2013;69:559–73.
28. Langlois F, Lim DST, Fleseriu M. Update on adrenal insufficiency: diagnosis and management in pregnancy. Curr Opin Endocrinol Diabetes Obes 2017;24:184–92.

29. Jung C, Ho JT, Torpy DJ, et al. A longitudinal study of plasma and urinary cortisol in pregnancy and postpartum. J Clin Endocrinol Metab 2011;96:1533–40.
30. Demey-Ponsart E, Foidart JM, Sulon J, et al. Serum CBG, free and total cortisol and circadian patterns of adrenal function in normal pregnancy. J Steroid Biochem 1982;16:165–9.
31. Ambroziak U, Kondracka A, Bartoszewicz Z, et al. The morning and late-night salivary cortisol ranges for healthy women may be used in pregnancy. Clin Endocrinol 2015;83:774–8.
32. Lopes LM, Francisco RP, Galletta MA, et al. Determination of nighttime salivary cortisol during pregnancy: comparison with values in non-pregnancy and Cushing's disease. Pituitary 2016;19:30–8.
33. Odagiri E, Ishiwatari N, Abe Y, et al. Hypercortisolism and the resistance to dexamethasone suppression during gestation. Endocrinol Jpn 1988;35:685–90.
34. Yang Q, Wang W, Liu C, et al. Compartmentalized localization of 11beta-HSD 1 and 2 at the feto-maternal interface in the first trimester of human pregnancy. Placenta 2016;46:63–71.
35. Okamoto E, Takagi T, Makino T, et al. Immunoreactive corticotropin-releasing hormone, adrenocorticotropin and cortisol in human plasma during pregnancy and delivery and postpartum. Horm Metab Res 1989;21:566–72.
36. Owens PC, Smith R, Brinsmead MW, et al. Postnatal disappearance of the pregnancy-associated reduced sensitivity of plasma cortisol to feedback inhibition. Life Sci 1987;41:1745–50.
37. Parksook WW, Porntharukchareon T, Sunthornyothin S. Desmopressin Stimulation Test in a Pregnant Patient with Cushing's Disease. AACE Clin Case Rep 2022;8:105–8.
38. Hamblin R, Coulden A, Fountas A, et al. The diagnosis and management of Cushing's syndrome in pregnancy. J Neuroendocrinol 2022;34:e13118.
39. Younes N, St-Jean M, Bourdeau I, et al. Endogenous Cushing's syndrome during pregnancy. Rev Endocr Metab Disord 2023;24:23–38.
40. Wagner J, Langlois F, Lim DST, et al. Hypercoagulability and Risk of Venous Thromboembolic Events in Endogenous Cushing's Syndrome: A Systematic Meta-Analysis. Front Endocrinol 2018;9:805.
41. Martinez GR, Martinez PA, Domingo del PC, et al. Cushing's syndrome in pregnancy. Laparoscopic adrenalectomy during pregnancy: the mainstay treatment. J Endocrinol Invest 2016;39:273–6.
42. Fleseriu M, Hashim IA, Karavitaki N, et al. Hormonal Replacement in Hypopituitarism in Adults: An Endocrine Society Clinical Practice Guideline. J Clin Endocrinol Metab 2016;101:3888–921.
43. Gheorghiu ML, Negreanu F, Fleseriu M. Updates in the Medical Treatment of Pituitary Adenomas. Horm Metab Res 2020;52:8–24.
44. Azzola A, Eastabrook G, Matsui D, et al. Adrenal Cushing Syndrome Diagnosed During Pregnancy: Successful Medical Management With Metyrapone. J Endocr Soc 2021;5:bvaa167.
45. Bass IR, Leiter A, Pozharny Y, et al. Cushing Disease Treated Successfully With Metyrapone During Pregnancy. AACE Clin Case Rep 2022;8:78–81.
46. Iioka M, Hayakawa T, Otsuki M, et al. A Rare Case of Placental Abruption and Postpartum Compression Fractures in Pregnancy With Cushing Syndrome. JCEM Case Rep 2023;1:luad128.
47. Ralser DJ, Strizek B, Kupczyk P, et al. Obstetric and Neonatal Outcome of Pregnancy in Carney Complex: A Case Report. Front Endocrinol 2020;11:296.

48. Takeuchi N, Imamura Y, Ishiwata K, et al. Cushing's syndrome in pregnancy in which laparoscopic adrenalectomy was safely performed by a retroperitoneal approach. IJU Case Rep 2023;6:415–8.
49. Zieleniewski W, Michalak R. A successful case of pregnancy in a woman with ACTH-independent Cushing's syndrome treated with ketoconazole and metyrapone. Gynecol Endocrinol 2017;33:349–52.
50. Berwaerts J, Verhelst J, Mahler C, et al. Cushing's syndrome in pregnancy treated by ketoconazole: case report and review of the literature. Gynecol Endocrinol 1999;13:175–82.
51. Boronat M, Marrero D, Lopez-Plasencia Y, et al. Successful outcome of pregnancy in a patient with Cushing's disease under treatment with ketoconazole during the first trimester of gestation. Gynecol Endocrinol 2011;27:675–7.
52. Kyriakos G, Farmaki P, Voutyritsa E, et al. Cushing's syndrome in pregnancy: a review of reported cases. Endokrynol Pol 2021;72:64–72.
53. Petersenn S, Fleseriu M, Casanueva FF, et al. Diagnosis and management of prolactin-secreting pituitary adenomas: a Pituitary Society international Consensus Statement. Nat Rev Endocrinol 2023;19:722–40.
54. Murillo NB, Ramacciotti CF, Fux-Otta C, et al. [Cushing's disease in pregnancy and treatment with cabergoline: obstetric and neonatal results]. Rev Fac Cien Med Univ Nac Cordoba 2023;80:55–8.
55. Nakhleh A, Saiegh L, Reut M, et al. Cabergoline treatment for recurrent Cushing's disease during pregnancy. Hormones (Basel) 2016;15:453–8.
56. Sek KS, Deepak DS, Lee KO. Use of cabergoline for the management of persistent Cushing's disease in pregnancy. BMJ Case Rep 2017;bcr2016217855.
57. Woo I, Ehsanipoor RM. Cabergoline therapy for Cushing disease throughout pregnancy. Obstet Gynecol 2013;122:485–7.

Hypercalcemia Associated with Pregnancy and Lactation

Yasaman Motlaghzadeh, MPH, MD[a], John P. Bilezikian, MD[b],
Deborah E. Sellmeyer, MD[a],*

KEYWORDS

- Hypercalcemia • 1,25 dihydroxyvitamin D • Pregnancy • PTHrP
- Hyperparathyroidism • Calcitriol • Lactation • Milk alkali

KEY POINTS

- Primary hyperparathyroidism (PHPT) is the primary etiology of hypercalcemia during pregnancy, most often due to a solitary parathyroid adenoma.
- While challenging, ruling out familial hypocalciuric hypercalcemia is important to avoid inappropriate parathyroidectomy.
- When conservative treatments prove ineffective in managing PHPT, parathyroidectomy during the second trimester is recommended.
- Many other nonparathyroid etiologies of hypercalcemia have been described associated with pregnancy and lactation.
- Medical treatment options for hypercalcemia during pregnancy are limited due to a lack of safety data.

INTRODUCTION

Pregnancy and lactation place significant demands on the maternal calciotropic system. Approximately 30 g of calcium and 20 g of phosphorus are required by the fetus at the end of a full-term gestation followed by even higher amounts needed during 6 months of lactation.[1] Many hormonal and physiologic adaptations help to meet these increased requirements. Hypercalcemia during pregnancy is uncommon because typically these physiologic adaptations are not associated with any changes in the maternal circulating concentration of calcium. However, when hypercalcemia occurs, a distinctly pathophysiological condition, adverse maternal and fetal consequences can result. A delay in recognition of hypercalcemia can occur if it is based on symptoms, because

[a] Division of Endocrinology, Gerontology and Metabolism, Department of Medicine, Stanford University School of Medicine, Palo Alto, CA, USA; [b] Division of Endocrinology, Department of Medicine, Columbia University, New York, USA
* Corresponding author. 300 Pasteur Drive, M/C 5103, Palo Alto, CA 94305.
E-mail address: dsellme@stanford.edu

Endocrinol Metab Clin N Am 53 (2024) 437–452
https://doi.org/10.1016/j.ecl.2024.05.006   endo.theclinics.com

they overlap with common symptoms associated with routine pregnancies. While primary hyperparathyroidism (PHPT) is the most common etiology of hypercalcemia during pregnancy, many other causes of hypercalcemia have been described as well. Early recognition of PHPT is important because if surgery is to be performed, it should be done during the second trimester. Medical treatment options are limited during pregnancy due to potential adverse effects of most pharmacologic therapies on fetal development. This review discusses the physiologic changes that occur during pregnancy and lactation, the etiologies of hypercalcemia that have been described during pregnancy and lactation, and the treatment strategies available.

CHANGES IN MINERAL METABOLISM DURING PREGNANCY AND LACTATION
Mineral and Hormonal Changes During Pregnancy

Maternal serum total calcium decreases during pregnancy due to hemodilution, although ionized calcium remains normal as do maternal phosphorus and magnesium levels. A standard normal range for serum calcium in pregnancy has not been established; however, due to hemodilution, albumin-adjusted calcium or ionized calcium should be used when assessing for hypercalcemia. During pregnancy, levels of active vitamin D (1,25-dihydroxyvitamin D or calcitriol) increase up to 5 fold due to increased activity of 1-alpha-hydroxylase in the maternal kidneys under the influence of parathyroid hormone-related peptide (PTHrP), estradiol, prolactin, and placental lactogen.[2] While the placenta also expresses this activating enzyme, the placenta appears to contribute minimally to maternal circulating calcitriol levels. Maternal parathyroid hormone (PTH) levels decline during pregnancy by as much as 30% during the first trimester with an increase to the middle of the normal range later in pregnancy. The early decrease in PTH is blunted or absent in the setting of calcium or vitamin D deficiency.[1] PTHrP increases progressively throughout gestation, likely from breast and placental sources. The exact role of PTHrP in maternal–fetal calcium metabolism is not fully understood. However, PTHrP may play a role in increasing calcitriol, regulating placental calcium transport, and potentially preventing excessive maternal bone resorption.[1,3]

Intestinal and Renal Changes During Pregnancy

By the 12th week of pregnancy, intestinal calcium absorption is doubled, well before the substantial increase in calcitriol which occurs during the third trimester. Other hormones including placental lactogen and prolactin may also contribute to increased calcium absorption.[2] Increased intestinal calcium absorption appears to be the primary mechanism by which fetal calcium needs are met. Concurrent with the increased calcium absorption, renal calcium excretion increases and can reach levels above the normal range. Fasting urine calcium is normal or low, demonstrating the hypercalciuria is due to increased intestinal absorption.[1] The absorptive hypercalciuria that occurs during pregnancy impedes differentiating familial hypocalciuric hypercalcemia from PHPT.

Calcium Metabolism During Lactation

Mobilization of calcium from the maternal skeleton due to increased PTHrP production by the breast as well as decreased estradiol levels appears to be the primary mechanism to meet the calcium needs of lactation.[1] Intestinal calcium absorption and calcitriol levels rapidly decrease to normal levels postpartum. Urinary calcium levels decrease, likely reflecting increased tubular reabsorption of calcium under the influence of PTHrP.

EFFECTS OF HYPERCALCEMIA ON MATERNAL AND FETAL OUTCOMES

Nonspecific manifestations of hypercalcemia such as nausea, vomiting, fatigue, myalgias/arthralgias, and constipation overlap with symptoms that occur during normal pregnancy, which can delay recognition of hypercalcemia. Hypercalcemia during pregnancy appears to be uncommon, but no systematically collected data are available. Historically, hypercalcemia during pregnancy, largely due to PHPT, has been associated with adverse maternal outcomes such as hyperemesis, nephrolithiasis, and pancreatitis as well as intrauterine fetal death, stillbirth, spontaneous abortion, and neonatal tetany with rates as high as 30% or more.[4,5] While prior series included women with more severe degrees of hypercalcemia, most [6–9] but not all[10] more recent series also show an increased risk of pre-eclampsia, preterm delivery, emergency cesarean section, fetal growth restriction, and neonatal intensive care unit admission. Maternal hypercalcemia can induce neonatal hypocalcemia by suppressing fetal parathyroid gland function. If left unaddressed, this condition can impair fetal growth and potentially lead to seizures, fetal or neonatal mortality.[11–13]

ETIOLOGIES OF HYPERCALCEMIA IN PREGNANCY AND LACTATION

The wide array of etiologies of hypercalcemia that have been reported associated with pregnancy and lactation are detailed below and summarized in **Box 1**.

Parathyroid Hormone-mediated Hypercalcemia

Primary hyperparathyroidism

PHPT, although uncommon in women of childbearing age, remains the most common cause of hypercalcemia during pregnancy. Hypercalcemia during pregnancy can result in acute pancreatitis, nephrolithiasis, renal damage, cardiac arrhythmias, peptic ulcers, and altered mental status.[14–17] Additionally, a minority of pregnant women with PHPT, estimated at less than 10%, may experience reduced bone density and skeletal fractures.[18–20] Among a cohort of 17 cases of PHPT during pregnancy, nearly half were incidentally diagnosed. Symptoms reported at the time of diagnosis included recurrent miscarriage, severe headaches, severe gestational hypertension, kidney stones, and severe nausea/vomiting.[21] A retrospective study covering a 16 year period 1999 to 2015 examined data from 13,792,544 deliveries, identifying 368 cases of hyperparathyroidism in pregnant women. Women with hyperparathyroidism faced higher risks of preterm delivery, pre-eclampsia, cesarean delivery, fetal growth restriction, and congenital anomalies in the neonates.[9]

Diagnosis and imaging. During pregnancy, the diagnosis of hyperparathyroidism is based on elevated albumin-adjusted serum calcium or serum ionized calcium levels, along with increased or inappropriately normal serum PTH levels.[22] Before confirming a diagnosis of PHPT, other potential causes of PTH-induced hypercalcemia, such as the use of lithium and hydrochlorothiazide or familial hypocalciuric hypercalcemia (FHH), should be ruled out. In nonpregnant individuals, determining the 24 hour calcium/creatinine clearance ratio (CCCR) is helpful in distinguishing between FHH and PHPT. Typically, this ratio is below 0.01 in 80% of nonpregnant individuals with FHH. However, about 20% of nonpregnant individuals with FHH exhibit CCCRs ranging between 0.01 and 0.02, overlapping with values observed in PHPT. Furthermore, increased urinary calcium excretion in pregnant women complicates the identification of hypocalciuria in those pregnant women with FHH. Thus, while a low CCCR can effectively rule out PHPT, levels greater than 0.01 have limited value in distinguishing between PHPT and FHH.[23,24] Genetic testing can help to identify

> **Box 1**
> **Etiologies of hypercalcemia that have been reported in association with pregnancy and lactation**
>
> PTH-mediated hypercalcemia
> - Primary hyperparathyroidism
> - Hereditary causes (MEN1, MEN2A, MEN4, hyperparathyroidism-jaw tumor syndrome, familial isolated primary hyperparathyroidism)
> - Parathyroid cancer
> - Familial hypocalciuric hypercalcemia (FHH)
> - Parathyromatosis.
> - Tertiary hyperparathyroidism
>
> Calcitriol (1,25 dihydroxyvitamin D)-mediated hypercalcemia
> - CYP24A1 gene mutations
> - Sarcoidosis
>
> PTHrP-mediated hypercalcemia
> - Mammary hyperplasia
> - Placental secretion
> - Neoplasm (uterine leiomyomas, ovarian carcinoma, pancreatic neuroendocrine tumors, renal cell carcinoma, and schistosomal bladder carcinoma)
> - Lactation
>
> Other malignancies (multiple myeloma, metastatic melanoma)
>
> Milk alkali syndrome
>
> Overtreatment of hypoparathyroidism
>
> Vitamin D toxicity
>
> Hereditary hyperphosphatasia
>
> Adrenal insufficiency due to postpartum pituitary failure.
>
> *Abbreviations:* CYP24A1, cytochrome P450 family 24 subfamily A member 1; MEN1, multiple endocrine neoplasia type 1; MEN2A, multiple endocrine neoplasia type 2A; MEN4, multiple endocrine neoplasia type 4; PTH, parathyroid hormone; PTHrP, parathyroid hormone-related peptide.

individuals with FHH, but the results may not be available in a timely manner to make diagnostic decisions during pregnancy.

Imaging modalities for PHPT during pregnancy are somewhat limited. Among these, ultrasonography, with a sensitivity of approximately 80% to 89%, is the most helpful in localizing hyperfunctioning parathyroid gland(s) before surgical intervention, particularly in cases where parathyroid adenoma is the primary etiology.[25–27] However, ultrasound sensitivity falls to 15%–35% in instances of multiglandular disease.[28] Detecting ectopic parathyroid lesions situated beyond the cervical region poses a substantial challenge using this imaging modality.[29]

Nuclear medicine imaging, particularly 99mTc-MIBI SPECT, can be useful in identifying ectopic parathyroid tissue, but the radioisotope crosses the placenta and it is a class C drug.[30] While studies indicate its seeming safety in pregnant individuals with hyperparathyroidism,[31–33] particularly when resulting exposure is less than 5 mGy, caution is necessary due to the potential risk of radiation exposure to the developing fetus. It is therefore not routinely employed during pregnancy. A 2016 committee opinion from the American College of Obstetricians and Gynecologists stated that fetal exposure below 5 mGy is considered safe during pregnancy.[34]

Computed tomography (CT) scans should be avoided during pregnancy because the radiation exposure is higher than 99mTc-MIBI.[21] While MRI may be useful in identifying ectopic parathyroid glands, it is not routinely used for evaluation of hyperparathyroidism during pregnancy and data on sensitivity of MRI to detect hyperfunctioning parathyroid glands during pregnancy are limited.

Hereditary causes. The hereditary etiologies of PHPT can manifest as components of syndromes, such as multiple endocrine neoplasia (MEN1, MEN2A, and MEN4) and hyperparathyroidism-jaw tumor syndrome, or may present independently as familial isolated PHPT.[35,36] These genetic variants tend to become evident at an earlier age than sporadic cases of PHPT and exhibit a higher prevalence among women of reproductive age. According to the current PHPT guidelines,[37] genetic testing is advised for individuals under 30 years, those presenting with multigland disease, individuals with a familial history of hypercalcemia or specific syndromes, and those patients diagnosed with atypical parathyroid adenoma or parathyroid carcinoma.

In a series comparing maternofetal outcomes in mothers with MEN 1 at the Royal Hobart Hospital from 1967 to 2018, maternal MEN 1 was linked to higher risks of gestational diabetes, hypertensive disorders, and lower neonatal birth weights compared to Australian averages. Miscarriage rates did not increase despite worsening hypercalcemia in the second trimester, and most pregnancies progressed without significant complications or interventions.[36]

Parathyroid cancer
Parathyroid carcinoma, a rare disorder in general, is even more uncommon during pregnancy.[38–46] Timely intervention is critical in managing parathyroid carcinoma, with survival largely dependent on achieving complete primary resection. However, recurrence rates range notably between 30% and 65%, with fewer than 5% of cases maintaining normocalcemic for more than 2 years following treatment.[38] Higher levels of serum calcium and PTH, larger tumor size, and presence of local neck symptoms should prompt consideration of this diagnosis.

Familial hypocalciuric hypercalcemia
FHH is a rare autosomal-dominant disorder in which there are mild-to-moderate, nonprogressive elevations in serum calcium and PTH levels accompanied by hypocalciuria. This condition arises from dysfunctional calcium-sensing receptors attributed to 3 identified genetic variants. Despite fewer than 10 reported cases of FHH during pregnancy, the actual incidence is likely to be greater as asymptomatic hypercalcemia would readily go undetected during pregnancy since serum calcium measurements are not routinely obtained.[23,24,47] FHH rarely poses significant complications to maternal health during pregnancy. However, it can result in fetal issues such as mild hypercalcemia, severe hypocalcemia, or neonatal severe hyperparathyroidism, depending on the genotype of the fetus.[48] Although differentiation between PHPT and FHH during pregnancy is a challenge, it is important because in FHH, surgery should not be pursued.

Parathyromatosis
Parathyromatosis refers to the presence of multiple benign hyperfunctioning parathyroid nodules scattered throughout the neck and mediastinum. There is a single documented case report of parathyromatosis occurring during pregnancy. In this instance, a 21 year old woman who had previously undergone a 3.5 gland parathyroidectomy experienced severe hyperemesis during her first trimester. Further investigation

revealed PHPT due to parathyromatosis. The symptomatic hypercalcemia was managed safely and effectively with cinacalcet during the third trimester.[49]

Tertiary hyperparathyroidism
Tertiary hyperparathyroidism is a consequence of prolonged secondary hyperparathyroidism. It emerges as a hypercalcemic state after relentless stimulation of parathyroid tissue and emergence of parathyroid tissue that is semiautonomous. One documented case of tertiary hyperparathyroidism was described in a pregnant woman with a history of a renal transplant. Throughout the pregnancy and postpartum period, the extent of the hypercalcemia was stable. The newborn displayed mild hypocalcemia after birth, necessitating treatment with intravenous calcium.[50]

Calcitriol-mediated Hypercalcemia

Cytochrome P450 family 24 subfamily A member 1 gene mutations
The cytochrome P450 family 24 subfamily A member 1 (CYP24A1) gene encodes a mitochondrial enzyme known as 24-hydroxylase, responsible for the inactivation of 1,25-dihydroxyvitamin D. Loss-of-function mutations within CYP24A1 can lead to an increase in the concentration of active vitamin D, which in turn can cause hypercalcemia, nephrolithiasis, and nephrocalcinosis. In pregnant women, this mutation appears to be associated with more hypercalcemia than is usually seen in nonpregnant adults.[51–58]

In a 2021 systematic review of 25 pregnancies with CYP24A1 mutations, 20 cases reported symptomatic hypercalcemia. The onset of hypercalcemia was usually in the second or third trimester, occurring around a median gestational age of 23 weeks. Pregnancy was associated with more severe clinical and biochemical features compared to nonpregnant individuals possessing similar CYP24A1 genetic variants. Pregnant women demonstrated significantly higher serum calcium levels at diagnosis than nonpregnant counterparts with matching genetic profiles.[59]

Sarcoidosis
Hypercalcemia and hypercalciuria can occur in sarcoidosis due to uncontrolled extrarenal synthesis of 1,25-dihydroxy vitamin D within the macrophages of the sarcoid granuloma. Two case reports have described sarcoidosis in the early postpartum period—one displaying hypercalciuria and the other presenting with hypercalcemia.[60,61]

Parathyroid Hormone-related Peptide-mediated Hypercalcemia

Mammary hyperplasia
Owing to the autonomous secretion of PTHrP by the mammary glands and placenta, which is independent of serum calcium levels, excessive physiologic secretion PTHrP can cause hypercalcemia.[62,63] Gestational gigantomastia, characterized by aberrant and disproportionate breast tissue growth during pregnancy, can lead to PTHrP-mediated hypercalcemia. Of note, 2 patients necessitated bilateral mastectomy due to this condition.[64,65]

During the 15th week of her pregnancy, another young woman presented with substantial breast enlargement and was diagnosed with severe hypercalcemia, exhibiting reduced PTH levels along with an elevated concentration of PTHrP. Treatment with bromocriptine effectively suppressed PTHrP production and restored serum calcium levels to a normal range.[66]

Placental secretion
There have been 2 reported cases documenting PTHrP-associated hypercalcemia, likely originating from the placenta. Following delivery, there was a prompt reduction

in serum calcium levels observed in both cases. Furthermore, in one of these instances, a transient episode of "hungry bone" syndrome occurred.[67,68]

Neoplasm

Hypercalcemia associated with neoplastic conditions is a rare occurrence in pregnant patients. Uterine leiomyomas,[69–72] ovarian carcinoma,[73–75] pancreatic neuroendocrine tumors,[76,77] renal cell carcinoma,[78] and schistosomal bladder carcinoma[79] have all been reported in hypercalcemic pregnant women. The majority of these documented cases appeared to be attributed to tumoral production of PTHrP.

Lactation

A patient with hypoparathyroidism experienced hypercalcemia accompanied by elevated PTHrP levels during lactation. The hypercalcemia in this case responded favorably to the discontinuation of calcium and calcitriol supplements. However, despite the resolution of hypercalcemia, the levels of PTHrP remained persistently elevated.[80]

Other Malignancies

Malignancies causing bone destruction leading to hypercalcemia can also present during pregnancy. Multiple myeloma and widely metastatic melanoma causing hypercalcemia during pregnancy have been described.[81–83]

Milk Alkali

There are multiple case reports of milk alkali syndrome occurring in women using high doses of calcium carbonate antacids to treat gastroesophageal reflux during pregnancy and the early postpartum period with serum calcium values as high as 25.2 mg/dL[84–89] as well as one case of neonatal hypocalcemic seizures in the offspring of a woman consuming up to 6 g of calcium per day during the last months of her pregnancy.[90] Both H2-blockers and proton-pump inhibitors are considered safe during pregnancy and are, thus, preferred alternatives for treatment of gastrointestinal reflux.[91]

Overtreatment of Hypoparathyroidism

The significant changes in mineral metabolism during pregnancy, particularly non-PTH stimulation of 1-alpha-hydroxylase activity, increased urine calcium excretion, and lower values of total serum calcium complicate management of hypoparathyroidism, placing women at risk for hypercalcemia during pregnancy and postpartum.[92–94] A recent series of pregnancy outcomes among 204 women with hypoparathyroidism demonstrated an increased risk of preterm birth, need for maternal blood transfusion, and congenital anomalies in the neonates.[95] While supplemental amounts of calcium and vitamin D may not change during pregnancy, half of the pregnant women with hypoparathyroidism in a separate series required more than a 20% adjustment, either increase or decrease, in the dose of their active vitamin D to maintain normocalcemia during pregnancy.[96] Frequent (every 3–4 weeks) monitoring of serum total and ionized calcium with adjustments, particularly in active vitamin D doses, is needed to prevent hypercalcemia during pregnancy and lactation in women with hypoparathyroidism.

Vitamin D Toxicity

Excessive maternal vitamin D ingestion has been reported to cause neonatal hypercalcemia lasting as long as 4 months.[97,98] Maternal serum vitamin D levels in these cases ranged from 50.8 to 143 ng/mL with maternal vitamin D intakes ranging from 4000 IU/day to 300,000 IU every other day during pregnancy. Interestingly, maternal calcium levels remained normal, although one mother was demonstrated to have nephrocalcinosis.

Hereditary Hyperphosphatasia (Juvenile Paget's Disease)

After delivery, the high calcium transfer by the placenta ceases which may lead to hypercalcemia in the setting of an underlying high bone turnover state such as has been described in a patient with hereditary hyperphosphatasia (Juvenile Paget's disease).[99]

Adrenal Insufficiency due to Postpartum Pituitary Failure

While rare, adrenal insufficiency can present with hypercalcemia. Acute loss of pituitary function in the early postnatal period due to pituitary hemorrhage (Sheehan's syndrome) or hypophysitis should be considered in a patient presenting with hypercalcemia postpartum, particularly as this is a life-threatening situation.[100–102]

TREATMENT OF HYPERCALCEMIA IN PREGNANCY
Hydration

Intravenous hydration is the mainstay of treatment of hypercalcemia in pregnancy. The addition of furosemide, which is a pregnancy category C drug, should be limited to women at risk of congestive heart failure as it may affect uteroplacental circulation.[103] Frequent and large volume hydration can be required to lower serum calcium to the levels typical of pregnancy which are lower than in the nonpregnant state due to lower albumin, increased volume of distribution, and higher glomerular filtration rate (GFR). Thus, hydration may be limited by requiring a frequent intravenous access and long duration of infusion.

Parathyroid Surgery

Given the potential adverse outcomes of hypercalcemia for both the mother and neonate, the current consensus remains that parathyroidectomy should be considered in pregnant women with PHPT.[104,105] There are no specific guidelines regarding what level of calcium can be monitored conservatively versus recommending surgical intervention during pregnancy; however, similar cut points as those used in nonpregnant individuals are often followed.[37] Optimally, parathyroidectomy is performed in the second trimester using a minimally invasive technique with localization with ultrasound rather than sestamibi with intraoperative PTH monitoring, although more extensive procedures may be needed in the setting of hereditary disorders characterized by multigland disease.[31] Regional anesthesia can be used if appropriate surgical and anesthesia expertise is available. For women with PHPT planning to conceive, surgery should be considered prior to conception. If women with PHPT are managed conservatively during pregnancy, their offspring should be monitored closely for potential hypocalcemia after delivery.

Cinacalcet

Cinacalcet crosses the placenta and is categorized as a category C medication.[106] The use of cinacalcet in pregnancies complicated by hyperparathyroidism is limited to case reports with transient neonatal hypocalcemia noted as an adverse event.[107,108]

Bisphosphonates

Bisphosphonates cross the placenta and, in animal studies, have been associated with decreased fetal growth, dental abnormalities, skeletal malformations, and, at high doses, prolonged parturition and fetal loss due to maternal hypocalcemia.[109,110]

Bisphosphonates are categorized as category C (alendronate, risedronate, ibandronate) or D (pamidronate, zoledronic acid) medications. Multiple case series of pregnancies in women with exposure to bisphosphonates demonstrated no increase in congenital malformations, but higher rates of neonatal complications, lower birth weight, shorter gestational age, and transient hypocalcemia in the newborns were observed.[111–114]

Calcitonin

Calcitonin does not cross the placenta and is a category C drug in pregnancy. There are a number of case reports where calcitonin was used to treat hyperparathyroidism during pregnancy; however, use is limited by short duration of action, lack of safety data, and tachyphylaxis.[115]

Glucocorticoids

Glucocorticoids are the preferred treatment for hypercalcemia due to elevated calcitriol or vitamin D toxicity; however, glucocorticoids potentially could be helpful for any cause of hypercalcemia during pregnancy as these agents would inhibit the pregnancy-related increase in intestinal calcium absorption and 1-alpha-hydroxylase activity. In animal studies, glucocorticoid administration during pregnancy causes cleft palate; human studies suggest there may be a small increase in cleft lip with or without cleft palate associated with use of glucocorticoids in the first trimester.[116] No increase in other adverse outcomes such as low birth weight, pre-eclampsia, or preterm birth have been consistently demonstrated. While data are limited, 2 studies suggest an increased risk of gestational diabetes among women receiving glucocorticoids during pregnancy.[116]

Denosumab

There are no human data regarding denosumab; however, animal studies show impaired mammary development among dams treated with denosumab with increased bone mass in the offspring and a high rate of neonatal mortality.[117] Denosumab is a category C drug and should be avoided in pregnancy given the very limited information available. The US Food and Drug Administration pregnancy category classifications for medications prescribed for hypercalcemia are summarized in **Table 1**.

Table 1 US Food and Drug Administration pregnancy category classifications for medications prescribed for hypercalcemia	
Drug	**Category**
Bisphosphonates	
Alendronate, risedronate, ibandronate	C
Pamidronate, zoledronic acid	D
Calcitonin	C
Cinacalcet	C
Denosumab	C
Furosemide	C
Glucocorticoids	C

SUMMARY

Hypercalcemia is uncommon in pregnancy but it can be associated with adverse maternal and fetal outcomes. Diagnosis may be a challenge as serum calcium is not routinely measured during pregnancy and symptoms overlap with those associated with pregnancy itself. PHPT is the most common etiology of hypercalcemia in pregnancy, although virtually every other cause of hypercalcemia has been described. Distinguishing PHPT from FHH remains a challenge but is critical to ensure timely intervention for PHPT and avoidance of unnecessary surgery in FHH. Medical management for hypercalcemia in pregnancy is limited as most agents are not advised for use in pregnant women. Inherited disorders such as MEN and calcium-sensing receptor mutations have implications for the offspring as well as the mother and require coordinated care between the adult, pediatric, and genetic teams.

CLINICS CARE POINTS

- During pregnancy, the diagnosis of PHPT is based on elevated albumin-adjusted serum calcium or serum ionized calcium levels, along with increased or inappropriately normal serum PTH levels.
- Distinguishing between PHPT and FHH is crucial for timely intervention in PHPT and avoiding unwarranted surgery in instances of FHH.
- In pregnancy, the CCCR may lack reliability. Therefore, if FHH is a consideration, DNA analysis and/or testing for hypercalcemia in family members should be considered.
- Imaging modalities in PHPT should be used cautiously in pregnancy due to radiation exposure and reserved exclusively for guiding the surgical approach for patients in whom parathyroidectomy is planned.
- Mild PHPT may be managed conservatively and with supportive care. If conservative treatments prove ineffective, the second trimester parathyroidectomy is recommended.
- If PTH is not elevated, evaluation for other causes of hypercalcemia is warranted as hypercalcemia due to a wide array of etiologies can occur in pregnancy.
- Medical options to manage hypercalcemia during pregnancy are limited, as medications for hypercalcemia have very limited data in pregnancy.

DISCLOSURE

The authors declare that they have no relevant disclosures.

REFERENCES

1. Kovacs CS. In: Feingold KR, et al, editors. Calcium and phosphate metabolism and related disorders during pregnancy and lactation. South Dartmouth (MA): Endotext; 2000.
2. Kovacs CS. Maternal Mineral and Bone Metabolism During Pregnancy, Lactation, and Post-Weaning Recovery. Physiol Rev 2016;96(2):449–547.
3. Cornish J, Callon KE, Nicholson GC, et al. Parathyroid hormone-related protein-(107-139) inhibits bone resorption in vivo. Endocrinology 1997;138(3):1299–304.
4. Malekar-Raikar S, Sinnott BP. Primary hyperparathyroidism in pregnancy-a rare cause of life-threatening hypercalcemia: case report and literature review. Case Rep Endocrinol 2011;2011:520516.
5. Schnatz PF, Thaxton S. Parathyroidectomy in the third trimester of pregnancy. Obstet Gynecol Surv 2005;60(10):672–82.

6. Rigg J, Gilbertson E, Barrett HL, et al. Primary Hyperparathyroidism in Pregnancy: Maternofetal Outcomes at a Quaternary Referral Obstetric Hospital, 2000 Through 2015. J Clin Endocrinol Metab 2019;104(3):721–9.
7. Arshad MF, Elamin A, Bennet W, et al. Abnormal Calcium Levels are Associated With Worse Maternal and Fetal Outcomes; Results From an Exploratory Study. J Clin Endocrinol Metab 2023;108(12):e1642–8.
8. Cassir G, Sermer C, Malinowski AK. Impact of Perinatal Primary Hyperparathyroidism on Maternal and Fetal and Neonatal Outcomes: Retrospective Case Series. J Obstet Gynaecol Can 2020;42(6):750–6.
9. Trahan MJ, Antinora C, Czuzoj-Shulman N, et al. Obstetrical and neonatal outcomes among pregnancies complicated by hyperparathyroidism. J Matern Fetal Neonatal Med 2023;36(1):2170748.
10. Hirsch D, Kopel V, Nadler V, et al. Pregnancy outcomes in women with primary hyperparathyroidism. J Clin Endocrinol Metab 2015;100(5):2115–22.
11. Cakir U, Alan S, Erdeve Ö, et al. Late neonatal hypocalcemic tetany as a manifestation of unrecognized maternal primary hyperparathyroidism. Turk J Pediatr 2013;55(4):438–40.
12. Korkmaz HA, Ozkan B, Terek D, et al. Neonatal seizure as a manifestation of unrecognized maternal hyperparathyroidism. J Clin Res Pediatr Endocrinol 2013; 5(3):206–8.
13. Razavi CR, Charitou M, Marzouk M. Maternal atypical parathyroid adenoma as a cause of newborn hypocalcemic tetany. Otolaryngol Head Neck Surg 2014; 151(6):1084–5.
14. Bansal S, Kaushik RM, Kaushik R, et al. Primary hyperparathyroidism presenting as severe hypercalcemia with acute pancreatitis in pregnancy. Gynecol Endocrinol 2020;36(5):469–72.
15. Lee CC, Chao AS, Chang YL, et al. Acute pancreatitis secondary to primary hyperparathyroidism in a postpartum patient: a case report and literature review. Taiwan J Obstet Gynecol 2014;53(2):252–5.
16. Richa CG, Saad KJ, Chaaban AK, et al. A rare case of hypercalcemia-induced pancreatitis in a first trimester pregnant woman. Endocrinol Diabetes Metab Case Rep 2018;2018:170175.
17. Tsai WH, Lee CC, Cheng SP, et al. Hyperparathyroidism presenting as hyperemesis and acute pancreatitis in pregnancy: A case report. Medicine (Baltimore) 2021;100(14):e25451.
18. Kohlmeier L, Marcus R. Calcium disorders of pregnancy. Endocrinol Metab Clin North Am 1995;24(1):15–39.
19. Mokrysheva NG, Eremkina AK, Mirnaya SS, et al. A Case of Pregnancy Complicated by Primary Hyperparathyroidism Due to a Parathyroid Adenoma. Am J Case Rep 2019;20:53–9.
20. Negishi H, Kobayashi M, Nishida R, et al. Primary hyperparathyroidism and simultaneous bilateral fracture of the femoral neck during pregnancy. J Trauma 2002;52(2):367–9.
21. DiMarco AN, Meeran K, Christakis I, et al. Seventeen Cases of Primary Hyperparathyroidism in Pregnancy: A Call for Management Guidelines. J Endocr Soc 2019;3(5):1009–21.
22. Pallan S, Rahman MO, Khan AA. Diagnosis and management of primary hyperparathyroidism. BMJ 2012;344:e1013.
23. Ghaznavi SA, Saad NM, Donovan LE. The Biochemical Profile of Familial Hypocalciuric Hypercalcemia and Primary Hyperparathyroidism during Pregnancy

and Lactation: Two Case Reports and Review of the Literature. Case Rep Endocrinol 2016;2016:2725486.

24. Jones AR, Hare MJ, Brown J, et al. Familial Hypocalciuric Hypercalcemia in Pregnancy: Diagnostic Pitfalls. JBMR Plus 2020;4(6):e10362.

25. Nafisi Moghadam R, Amlelshahbaz AP, Namiranian N, et al. Comparative Diagnostic Performance of Ultrasonography and 99mTc-Sestamibi Scintigraphy for Parathyroid Adenoma in Primary Hyperparathyroidism; Systematic Review and Meta- Analysis. Asian Pac J Cancer Prev 2017;18(12):3195–200.

26. Salhi H, Bouziane T, Maaroufi M, et al. Primary hyperparathyroidism: Correlation between cervical ultrasound and MIBI scan. Ann Afr Med 2022;21(2):161–4.

27. Vitetta GM, Neri P, Chiecchio A, et al. Role of ultrasonography in the management of patients with primary hyperparathyroidism: retrospective comparison with technetium-99m sestamibi scintigraphy. J Ultrasound 2014;17(1):1–12.

28. Sepahdari AR, Bahl M, Harari A, et al. Predictors of Multigland Disease in Primary Hyperparathyroidism: A Scoring System with 4D-CT Imaging and Biochemical Markers. AJNR Am J Neuroradiol 2015;36(5):987–92.

29. Abusabeib A, Bhat H, El Ansari W, et al. Right ectopic paraesophageal parathyroid adenoma with refractory hypercalcemia in pregnancy: A case report and review of the literature. Int J Surg Case Rep 2020;77:229–34.

30. Gilbert WM, Newman PS, Eby-Wilkens E, et al. Technetium Tc 99m rapidly crosses the ovine placenta and intramembranous pathway. Am J Obstet Gynecol 1996;175(6):1557–62.

31. McMullen TP, Learoyd DL, Williams DC, et al. Hyperparathyroidism in pregnancy: options for localization and surgical therapy. World J Surg 2010;34(8):1811–6.

32. Saad AF, Pacheco LD, Costantine MM. Management of ectopic parathyroid adenoma in pregnancy. Obstet Gynecol 2014;124(2 Pt 2 Suppl 1):478–80.

33. Schaefer C, Meister R, Wentzeck R, et al. Fetal outcome after technetium scintigraphy in early pregnancy. Reprod Toxicol 2009;28(2):161–6.

34. American College of, O. and P. Gynecologists' Committee on Obstetric. Committee Opinion No. 656: Guidelines for Diagnostic Imaging During Pregnancy and Lactation. Obstet Gynecol 2016;127(2):e75–80.

35. Casteras A, Darder L, Zafon C, et al. Brown tumor of the jaw after pregnancy and lactation in a MEN1 patient. Endocrinol Diabetes Metab Case Rep 2016; 2016.

36. Hogg P, Thompson M, Burgess J. The clinical expression and impact of multiple endocrine neoplasia 1 during pregnancy. Clin Endocrinol (Oxf) 2020;93(4):429–38.

37. Bilezikian JP, Khan AA, Silverberg SJ, et al. Evaluation and Management of Primary Hyperparathyroidism: Summary Statement and Guidelines from the Fifth International Workshop. J Bone Miner Res 2022;37(11):2293–314.

38. Palmieri-Sevier A, Palmieri GM, Baumgartner CJ, et al. Case report: long-term remission of parathyroid cancer: possible relation to vitamin D and calcitriol therapy. Am J Med Sci 1993;306(5):309–12.

39. Hess HM, Dickson J, Fox HE. Hyperfunctioning parathyroid carcinoma presenting as acute pancreatitis in pregnancy. J Reprod Med 1980;25(2):83–7.

40. Parham GP, Orr JW. Hyperparathyroidism secondary to parathyroid carcinoma in pregnancy. A case report. J Reprod Med 1987;32(2):123–5.

41. Paul RG, Elston MS, Gill AJ, et al. Hypercalcaemia due to parathyroid carcinoma presenting in the third trimester of pregnancy. Aust N Z J Obstet Gynaecol 2012; 52(2):204–7.

42. Panchani R, Varma T, Goyal A, et al. Parathyroid carcinoma masquerading as morning sickness in pregnancy. Indian J Endocrinol Metab 2013;17(Suppl 1): S198–200.
43. Nadarasa K, Bailey M, Chahal H, et al. The use of cinacalcet in pregnancy to treat a complex case of parathyroid carcinoma. Endocrinol Diabetes Metab Case Rep 2014;2014:140056.
44. Baretic M, Tomić Brzac H, Dobrenić M, et al. Parathyroid carcinoma in pregnancy. World J Clin Cases 2014;2(5):151–6.
45. Gumber L, Sivasankaran K, Khan SMS. Parathyroid carcinoma presenting with ventricular bigeminy in pregnancy. BMJ Case Rep 2022;15(2):e247069.
46. Dematapitiya C, Perera C, Pathmanathan S, et al. Parathyroid carcinoma during pregnancy: a novel pathogenic CDC73 mutation - a case report. BMC Endocr Disord 2022;22(1):259.
47. Powell BR, Buist NR. Late presenting, prolonged hypocalcemia in an infant of a woman with hypocalciuric hypercalcemia. Clin Pediatr (Phila) 1990;29(4):241–3.
48. Cooper MS. Disorders of calcium metabolism and parathyroid disease. Best Pract Res Clin Endocrinol Metabol 2011;25(6):975–83.
49. Edling KL, Korenman SG, Janzen C, et al. A pregnant dilemma: primary hyperparathyroidism due to parathyromatosis in pregnancy. Endocr Pract 2014;20(2): e14–7.
50. Fromm GA, Labarrere CA, Ramirez J, et al. Hypercalcaemia in pregnancy in a renal transplant recipient with secondary hyperparathyroidism. Case report. Br J Obstet Gynaecol 1990;97(11):1049–53.
51. Hedberg F, Pilo C, Wikner J, et al. Three Sisters With Heterozygous Gene Variants of CYP24A1: Maternal Hypercalcemia, New-Onset Hypertension, and Neonatal Hypoglycemia. J Endocr Soc 2019;3(2):387–96.
52. Arnold N, O'Toole V, Huynh T, et al. Intractable hypercalcaemia during pregnancy and the postpartum secondary to pathogenic variants in CYP24A1. Endocrinol Diabetes Metab Case Rep 2019;2019:190114.
53. Kwong WT, Fehmi SM. Hypercalcemic Pancreatitis Triggered by Pregnancy With a CYP24A1 Mutation. Pancreas 2016;45(6):e31–2.
54. Pilz S, Theiler-Schwetz V, Pludowski P, et al. Hypercalcemia in Pregnancy Due to CYP24A1 Mutations: Case Report and Review of the Literature. Nutrients 2022; 14(12):2518.
55. Romasovs A, Jaunozola L, Berga-Švītiņa E, et al. Hypercalcemia and CYP24A1 Gene Mutation Diagnosed in the 2nd Trimester of a Twin Pregnancy: A Case Report. Am J Case Rep 2021;22:e931116.
56. Lemaitre M, Lionet A, Fages V, et al. Case report: Non-PTH-dependent hypercalcemia in pregnancy: Consider CYP24A1 mutations. Ann Endocrinol (Paris) 2023;84(6):758–60.
57. Griffin TP, Joyce CM, Alkanderi S, et al. Biallelic CYP24A1 variants presenting during pregnancy: clinical and biochemical phenotypes. Endocr Connect 2020;9(6):530–41.
58. Woods GN, Saitman A, Gao H, et al. A Young Woman With Recurrent Gestational Hypercalcemia and Acute Pancreatitis Caused by CYP24A1 Deficiency. J Bone Miner Res 2016;31(10):1841–4.
59. Cappellani D, Brancatella A, Morganti R, et al. Hypercalcemia due to CYP24A1 mutations: a systematic descriptive review. Eur J Endocrinol 2021;186(2): 137–49.
60. Subramanian P, Chinthalapalli H, Krishnan M, et al. Pregnancy and sarcoidosis: an insight into the pathogenesis of hypercalciuria. Chest 2004;126(3):995–8.

61. Wilson-Holt N. Post partum presentation of hypercalcaemic sarcoidosis. Post-grad Med J 1985;61(717):627–8.
62. Dobnig H, Kainer F, Stepan V, et al. Elevated parathyroid hormone-related pep-tide levels after human gestation: relationship to changes in bone and mineral metabolism. J Clin Endocrinol Metab 1995;80(12):3699–707.
63. Lippuner K, Zehnder HJ, Casez JP, et al. PTH-related protein is released into the mother's bloodstream during lactation: evidence for beneficial effects on maternal calcium-phosphate metabolism. J Bone Miner Res 1996;11(10): 1394–9.
64. Van Heerden JA, Gharib H, Jackson IT. Pseudohyperparathyroidism secondary to gigantic mammary hypertrophy. Arch Surg 1988;123(1):80–2.
65. Moazzami B, Chaichian S, Farahvash MR, et al. A Rare Case of Gestational Gi-gantomastia with Hypercalcemia: The Challenges of Management and Follow up. J Reprod Infertil 2016;17(4):243–6.
66. Winter EM, Appelman-Dijkstra NM. Parathyroid Hormone-Related Protein-Induced Hypercalcemia of Pregnancy Successfully Reversed by a Dopamine Agonist. J Clin Endocrinol Metab 2017;102(12):4417–20.
67. Eller-Vainicher C, Ossola MW, Beck-Peccoz P, et al. PTHrP-associated hypercal-cemia of pregnancy resolved after delivery: a case report. Eur J Endocrinol 2012;166(4):753–6.
68. Modarressi T, Levine MA, Tchou J, et al. Gestational Gigantomastia Complicated by PTHrP-Mediated Hypercalcemia. J Clin Endocrinol Metab 2018;103(9): 3124–30.
69. Kropf J, Vo M, Cheyney S, et al. Hypercalcemia Resulting from Necrotizing Leio-myoma in a Pregnant Female. Am J Case Rep 2020;21:e923412.
70. Tarnawa E, Sullivan S, Underwood P, et al. Severe hypercalcemia associated with uterine leiomyoma in pregnancy. Obstet Gynecol 2011;117(2 Pt 2):473–6.
71. Rahil A, Khan FY. Humoral hypercalcemic crisis in a pregnant woman with uter-ine leiomyoma. J Emerg Trauma Shock 2012;5(1):87–9.
72. Sobey N, Raubenheimer L. Cystic pelvi-abdominal mass in pregnancy: An un-common presentation of a subserosal leiomyoma. SA J Radiol 2019;23(1):1683.
73. Hwang CS, Park SY, Yu SH, et al. Hypercalcemia induced by ovarian clear cell carcinoma producing all transcriptional variants of parathyroid hormone-related peptide gene during pregnancy. Gynecol Oncol 2006;103(2):740–4.
74. McCormick TC, Muffly T, Lu G, et al. Aggressive small cell carcinoma of the ovary, hypercalcemic type with hypercalcemia in pregnancy, treated with con-servative surgery and chemotherapy. Int J Gynecol Cancer 2009;19(8): 1339–41.
75. Nelsen LL, Muirhead DM, Bell MC. Ovarian small cell carcinoma, hypercalcemic type exhibiting a response to high-dose chemotherapy. S D Med 2010;63(11): 375–7.
76. Ghazi AA, Boustani I, Amouzegar A, et al. Postpartum hypercalcemia second-ary to a neuroendocrine tumor of pancreas; a case report and review of litera-ture. Iran J Med Sci 2011;36(3):217–21.
77. Abraham P, Ralston SH, Hewison M, et al. Presentation of a PTHrP-secreting pancreatic neuroendocrine tumour, with hypercalcaemic crisis, pre-eclampsia, and renal failure. Postgrad Med J 2002;78(926):752–3.
78. Usta IM, Chammas M, Khalil AM. Renal cell carcinoma with hypercalcemia complicating a pregnancy: case report and review of the literature. Eur J Gynae-col Oncol 1998;19(6):584–7.

79. Lortholary O, Babinet P, Mechali D, et al. Paraneoplastic hypercalcaemia in association with schistosomal bladder cancer. Br J Urol 1989;64(5):550–1.
80. Mather KJ, Chik CL, Corenblum B. Maintenance of serum calcium by parathyroid hormone-related peptide during lactation in a hypoparathyroid patient. J Clin Endocrinol Metab 1999;84(2):424–7.
81. Ceusters E, Fontaine C, Laubach C, et al. Hypercalcaemia due to metastatic melanoma during pregnancy. J Obstet Gynaecol 2000;20(2):195.
82. McIntosh J, Lauer J, Gunatilake R, et al. Multiple myeloma presenting as hypercalcemic pancreatitis during pregnancy. Obstet Gynecol 2014;124(2 Pt 2 Suppl 1):461–3.
83. Smith D, Stevens J, Quinn J, et al. Myeloma presenting during pregnancy. Hematol Oncol 2014;32(1):52–5.
84. Bailey CS, Weiner JJ, Gibby OM, et al. Excessive calcium ingestion leading to milk-alkali syndrome. Ann Clin Biochem 2008;45(Pt 5):527–9.
85. D'Souza R, Gandhi S, Fortinsky KJ, et al. Calcium carbonate intoxication in pregnancy: the return of the milk-alkali syndrome. J Obstet Gynaecol Can 2013;35(11):976–7.
86. Picolos MK, Sims CR, Mastrobattista JM, et al. Milk-alkali syndrome in pregnancy. Obstet Gynecol 2004;104(5 Pt 2):1201–4.
87. Tran HA. Life-threatening milk-alkali syndrome resulting from antacid ingestion during pregnancy. Med J Aust 2005;182(12):654, author reply 655.
88. Ennen CS, Magann EF. Milk-alkali syndrome presenting as acute renal insufficiency during pregnancy. Obstet Gynecol 2006;108(3 Pt 2):785–6.
89. Murphy ML, Mattingly MJ, Meisner CT. Severe Hypercalcemia in a Postpartum Patient. J Emerg Med 2016;51(4):e93–5.
90. Borkenhagen JF, Connor EL, Stafstrom CE. Neonatal hypocalcemic seizures due to excessive maternal calcium ingestion. Pediatr Neurol 2013;48(6):469–71.
91. Weiner CP, Buhimschi C. Drugs for pregnant and lactating women. 2nd edition. Philadelphia, PA: Elsevier Inc; 2009.
92. Cundy T, Haining SA, Guilland-Cumming DF, et al. Remission of hypoparathyroidism during lactation: evidence for a physiological role for prolactin in the regulation of vitamin D metabolism. Clin Endocrinol (Oxf) 1987;26(6):667–74.
93. Wright AD, Joplin GF, Dixon HG. Post-partum hypercalcaemia in treated hypoparathyroidism. Br Med J 1969;1(5635):23–5.
94. Caplan RH, Beguin EA. Hypercalcemia in a calcitriol-treated hypoparathyroid woman during lactation. Obstet Gynecol 1990;76(3 Pt 2):485–9.
95. Hochberg A, Pare A, Badeghiesh AM, et al. Pregnancy, delivery and neonatal outcomes among women with hypoparathyroidism-A population-based study. Clin Endocrinol (Oxf) 2023;99(6):525–32.
96. Hartogsohn EAR, Khan AA, Kjaersulf LU, et al. Changes in treatment needs of hypoparathyroidism during pregnancy and lactation: A case series. Clin Endocrinol (Oxf) 2020;93(3):261–8.
97. Karacan Kucukali G, Keskin M, Savaş Erdeve Ş, et al. Perinatal outcomes of high-dose vitamin D administration in the last trimester. Turk J Obstet Gynecol 2021;18(2):159–62.
98. Reynolds A, O'Connell SM, Kenny LC, et al. Transient neonatal hypercalcaemia secondary to excess maternal vitamin D intake: too much of a good thing. BMJ Case Rep 2017;2017. bcr2016219043.
99. Chosich N, Long F, Wong R, et al. Post-partum hypercalcemia in hereditary hyperphosphatasia (juvenile Paget's disease). J Endocrinol Invest 1991;14(7):591–7.

100. Bigos ST, Carnes TD. Isolated ACTH deficiency presenting as severe hypercalcemia. Am J Med Sci 1982;284(1):24–30.
101. Richtsmeier AJ, Henry RA, Bloodworth JM, et al. Lymphoid hypophysitis with selective adrenocorticotropic hormone deficiency. Arch Intern Med 1980;140(9): 1243–5.
102. Vasikaran SD, Tallis GA, Braund WJ. Secondary hypoadrenalism presenting with hypercalcaemia. Clin Endocrinol (Oxf) 1994;41(2):261–4.
103. Kaye AB, Bhakta A, Moseley AD, et al. Review of Cardiovascular Drugs in Pregnancy. J Womens Health (Larchmt) 2019;28(5):686–97.
104. Appelman-Dijkstra NM, Pilz S. Approach to the Patient: Management of Parathyroid Diseases Across Pregnancy. J Clin Endocrinol Metab 2023;108(6):1505–13.
105. Bollerslev J, Rejnmark L, Zahn A, et al. European Expert Consensus on Practical Management of Specific Aspects of Parathyroid Disorders in Adults and in Pregnancy: Recommendations of the ESE Educational Program of Parathyroid Disorders. Eur J Endocrinol 2022;186(2):R33–63.
106. Available at. https://www.accessdata.fda.gov/drugsatfda_docs/label/2011/021688s017lbl.pdf.
107. Horjus C, Groot I, Telting D, et al. Cinacalcet for hyperparathyroidism in pregnancy and puerperium. J Pediatr Endocrinol Metab 2009;22(8):741–9.
108. Rubin MR, Silverberg SJ. Use of Cinacalcet and (99m)Tc-sestamibi Imaging During Pregnancy. J Endocr Soc 2017;1(9):1156–9.
109. French AE, Kaplan N, Lishner M, et al. Taking bisphosphonates during pregnancy. Can Fam Physician 2003;49:1281–2.
110. Stathopoulos IP, Liakou CG, Katsalira A, et al. The use of bisphosphonates in women prior to or during pregnancy and lactation. Hormones (Athens) 2011; 10(4):280–91.
111. Djokanovic N, Klieger-Grossmann C, Koren G. Does treatment with bisphosphonates endanger the human pregnancy? J Obstet Gynaecol Can 2008;30(12): 1146–8.
112. Machairiotis N, Ntali G, Kouroutou P, et al. Clinical evidence of the effect of bisphosphonates on pregnancy and the infant. Horm Mol Biol Clin Investig 2019;40(2).
113. Abdul Ghani SF, Wright M, Paramo JG, et al. Three bisphosphonate ligands improve the water solubility of quantum dots. Faraday Discuss 2014;175: 153–69.
114. Green SB, Pappas AL. Effects of maternal bisphosphonate use on fetal and neonatal outcomes. Am J Health Syst Pharm 2014;71(23):2029–36.
115. Ali DS, Dandurand K, Khan AA. Primary Hyperparathyroidism in Pregnancy: Literature Review of the Diagnosis and Management. J Clin Med 2021;10(13): 2956.
116. Bandoli G, Palmsten K, Forbess Smith CJ, et al. A Review of Systemic Corticosteroid Use in Pregnancy and the Risk of Select Pregnancy and Birth Outcomes. Rheum Dis Clin North Am 2017;43(3):489–502.
117. Okamatsu N, Sakai N, Karakawa A, et al. Biological effects of anti-RANKL antibody administration in pregnant mice and their newborns. Biochem Biophys Res Commun 2017;491(3):614–21.

Bone Metabolism, Bone Mass, and Bone Structure During Pregnancy and Lactation

Normal Physiology and Pregnancy and Lactation-Associated Osteoporosis

Adi Cohen, MD, MHS

KEYWORDS

- Pregnancy and lactation-associated osteoporosis • Premenopausal osteoporosis
- Bone mineral density • Vertebral fracture • Osteoporosis treatment

KEY POINTS

- Normal pregnancy and lactation are states of high calcium demand and are associated with substantial changes in bone metabolism and bone density.
- Pregnancy and lactation-associated osteoporosis (PLO; sometimes abbreviated as pregnancy associated osteoporosis/lactation associated osteoporosis [PAO/LAO] or pregnancy and lactation associated osteoporosis [PLAO]) is a term used to describe an early onset osteoporosis presentation with fragility fractures that occur in the context of the bone mass and metabolism changes associated with pregnancy and lactation.
- The majority of cases identified as PLO include vertebral fracture(s); symptom onset is usually during lactation, rather than during pregnancy. Very low bone mineral density (BMD) by dual energy x-ray absorptiometry (DXA) and volumetric/structural bone deficits have been documented.

INTRODUCTION

This article will review bone metabolism, bone mass, and bone structure changes expected during and after pregnancy and lactation, as well as the condition of pregnancy and lactation-associated osteoporosis (PLO)—a presentation with fragility fracture(s) in the context of these physiologic changes. Clinical implications of physiologic bone changes will be addressed, as will specific management considerations that apply to premenopausal women with PLO.

Division of Endocrinology, Department of Medicine, Columbia University, College of Physicians & Surgeons, 180 Fort Washington Avenue, HP9-910, New York, NY 10032, USA
E-mail address: ac1044@columbia.edu

Endocrinol Metab Clin N Am 53 (2024) 453–470
https://doi.org/10.1016/j.ecl.2024.05.003
0889-8529/24/© 2024 Elsevier Inc. All rights reserved, including those for text and data mining, AI training, and similar technologies.

endo.theclinics.com

BONE CHANGES DURING PREGNANCY AND POSTPARTUM: NORMAL PHYSIOLOGY

Normal pregnancy and lactation are states of high calcium demand due to fetal and infant calcium needs. Several processes—including hormonal changes, changes in calcium absorption and renal calcium handling, and skeletal demineralization—meet these needs during normal reproduction.

Bone and Mineral Metabolism

Physiologic changes in mineral metabolism during pregnancy and lactation are outlined in several detailed reviews[1–3] and are summarized here.

During pregnancy, a high estrogen state also associated with expanded intravascular volume and a lower albumin level, serum total calcium declines but ionized calcium remains unchanged. Parathyroid hormone (PTH) declines while PTH-related protein (PTHrp; likely from breast and placental production) rises over the course of pregnancy.[2] Calcitriol (1,25(OH)$_2$ vitamin D) production rises dramatically,[4] leading to a doubling of calcium absorption that begins early in pregnancy.[2] An absorptive hypercalciuria can occur in this context and may contribute to increased renal stone risk during this time. Serum markers of bone turnover increase, peaking in the third trimester.[2,5,6] One bone biopsy study, evaluating women in early (n = 15) and late (n = 13) pregnancy in comparison to nonpregnant controls, showed increased bone resorption in early pregnancy (8–10 weeks gestation) and evidence of increased bone formation in late pregnancy (39–40 weeks gestation).[7]

After delivery,[2,8] estradiol levels fall and calcitriol levels and gastrointestinal calcium absorption return to nonpregnant levels. *During lactation*,[1,2,8] ionized calcium and phosphate levels rise as these minerals are mobilized from bone. A low-estrogen state contributes to the stimulation of bone resorption—but the process is largely driven by PTHrp. PTH is suppressed while PTHrp, produced by breast tissue, mediates calcium mobilization from bone[3] as well as renal calcium conservation.[2] Unlike other states of high bone turnover and bone loss, urinary calcium is generally reduced during this time, as the mobilized calcium is moved to breast milk. Serum markers of resorption and formation increase during lactation, peaking at 4 to 6 months postpartum in women who breastfed for 6 months or more.[2,9] Histomorphometric data are available in animal models; both osteoclast-mediated bone resorption (primarily in trabecular bone) and osteocytic osteolysis (in trabecular and cortical bone) contribute to mineral mobilization.[2,3,10]

During and postweaning, the process of increased bone resorption ceases in the context of resumption of menses, rising estradiol levels, lowered calcium demand and declining PTHrp. A process of remineralization and a shift toward bone formation ensues.[3] In animal models, bone formation markers rise while bone resorption markers decline, and histomorphometry reveals evidence of osteoclast apoptosis and increased bone formation as well as a shift to anabolic activity of osteocytes in the lacunar space.[2,3,11,12] Data from postpartum women who weaned at less than 6 months postpartum also show a rapid decline in the bone resorption marker, N-telopeptide (urine), with more gradual decline in the bone formation marker, osteocalcin (serum), over 20 months of follow-up.[9]

In summary, during pregnancy, increased calcium needs are largely met by a state of enhanced gastrointestinal calcium absorption, while during lactation, calcium needs are largely met by maternal skeletal bone resorption/demineralization. During the postweaning recovery and remineralization period, the balance of bone remodeling shifts to bone formation.

Bone Mineral Density and Bone Structure Changes During Pregnancy and Postpartum

Demineralization and the resulting maternal bone loss meet some of the fetal and infant calcium needs during normal reproduction. Thus, pregnancy and lactation are both associated with declines in bone mineral density (BMD), followed by recovery. Data on bone mass and structure changes in human pregnancy, postpartum, and during lactation will be summarized below. Studies in rodent models also contribute to our understanding of skeletal structural changes during this time, but the differences from humans in terms of metabolic adaptations,[2] continuing bone growth during reproduction, as well as relative calcium demand/litter size should be kept in mind when interpreting results.

During pregnancy, changes in bone mass have been documented in studies that have compared prepregnancy and postpregnancy assessments of BMD in women. These have shown moderate 3% to 5% declines[5,6,13,14] to no change[15] in BMD by DXA at the spine and other sites over pregnancy. A study assessing forearm BMD by DXA in each trimester of pregnancy showed declines at the ultradistal site, a site rich in trabecular bone, in comparison to nonpregnant controls.[14] Changes in bone structure over pregnancy have been assessed in rodent models and in a high-resolution peripheral quantitative computed tomographic (HR-pQCT) study of pregnant women. Studies in rodent models document trabecular thinning and reduced connectivity but increased cortical thickness over pregnancy.[16,17] In contrast, an HR-pQCT study of pregnant women imaged at 14 to 16 weeks gestation and 34 to 36 weeks gestation and compared to longitudinally followed nonpregnant controls, showed declines in total and cortical volumetric bone density (vBMD) and cortical thickness, but an increase in cortical perimeter at the tibia, with no significant changes at the radius, over pregnancy.[18] These data suggest that there may be compartment and site-specific bone structural changes over human pregnancy.

In postpartum women who choose not to breastfeed or who breastfeed for 0 to 1 month, stable BMD or small increases in BMD have been observed in observational studies over 6 to 12 months postpartum.[19–21] Increases during this time may reflect recovery of pregnancy-related bone loss. Calcium supplementation may have a beneficial effect in this context: In a 6 month randomized study (n = 81) of calcium supplementation (1 g elemental calcium per day as calcium carbonate) versus placebo, calcium supplementation was associated with a significant gain in lumbar spine BMD versus placebo (+2.2% vs +0.4%; $P < .05$) in nonlactating postpartum women.[19]

In postpartum women who choose to breastfeed for 6 months or longer, substantial areal BMD declines of 3% to 10% have been documented[1,2,19–22] at the spine and femoral neck in many studies utilizing DXA assessments. Calcium supplementation does not change this BMD trajectory. In a 6 month randomized study of calcium supplementation (1 g elemental calcium per day as calcium carbonate) versus placebo in 87 lactating postpartum women, lumbar spine bone loss averaged 4% to 5% at 6 months and did not differ between the groups.[19] It is possible that exercise could affect this trajectory[16]—one study of exclusively breastfeeding women documented significantly less spine DXA BMD loss between 3 and 21 weeks postpartum in a group randomized to a core strengthening and aerobic exercise intervention versus controls (mean ± SE: −7.02 ± 0.6% vs −4.8 ± 0.3%; $P < .05$).[23] This is consistent with the findings of similar effects of tibial mechanical loading in rats studied during the lactation period.[24]

Changes in vBMD and bone structure in the postpartum period have also been evaluated in 2 longitudinal HR-pQCT studies in healthy postpartum women.[25,26] In an

18 month study of 81 postpartum women, classified by lactation duration, those who breastfed for greater than 4 months had significant declines in both cortical and trabecular vBMD, and cortical and trabecular thickness, at the tibia.[26] In a study of 58 postpartum women assessed by HR-pQCT at the radius and tibia, decreases in trabecular number and mineralization density and increases in trabecular separation as well as cortical porosity were documented between the postpartum baseline and a second timepoint at the cessation of exclusive breastfeeding (median timing 5 months postpartum).[25] Studies of rat bone microstructure during this time document preferential trabecular bone loss, with large declines in trabecular number, thickness, and connectivity (>50% for several parameters),[16,17] and smaller declines in cortical area and thickness (14%–15%) during a first cycle of reproduction. De Bakker and colleagues also showed that the first reproductive cycle was associated with more bone loss than subsequent reproductive cycles.[17]

Assessments utilizing finite element analyses of imaging data to determine whole bone stiffness (of the proximal tibia, studied longitudinally)[17] or mechanical testing (of vertebra and femur, studied at different timepoints)[27] provide evidence of markedly reduced bone strength associated with lactation in rodent models—suggesting that the BMD changes seen in humans may also be associated with decreased bone strength. However, even given the large physiologic changes in bone density associated with breastfeeding in postpartum women, fractures during this period are thought to be very rare.

Studies with follow-up periods of at least 12 months postpartum document a change in BMD trajectory around 6 months, with bone mass increase and recovery after this timepoint, even with continued lactation.[1,2,20–22] In the setting of continued lactation, this change in trajectory is likely to relate to evolving calcium demand for milk production as the infant diet changes to include more solid food. Duration of lactation and duration of postpartum amenorrhea have both been associated with the postpartum BMD trajectory.[20–22] Calcium supplementation appears to aid the bone recovery process postweaning: In 76 postpartum breastfeeding women studied in the context of weaning between 6 and 12 months postpartum, the group randomized to calcium carbonate 1 g/d had significantly more BMD increase at the lumbar spine (mean $\pm$ SE, adjusted analysis: $+5.9 \pm 0.3\%$ vs $+4.4 \pm 0.3\%$; $P < .05$) over this 6 month period.[19] Mechanical loading has also been studied in this context,[2,16,24] but it remains unclear whether exercise or mechanical loading can alter the recovery process.

Several studies document a site-specific pattern of BMD recovery with full recovery of spine bone mass that returns to or exceeds the postpartum baseline by 12 months postpartum, but incomplete (or delayed) recovery at the femoral neck, which remains below the postpartum baseline at the end of the follow-up period.[20–22,28] HR-pQCT studies examining the postpartum bone recovery period also note lasting structural changes: one study found that tibial cortical vBMD and trabecular thickness remained lower versus baseline at the 18 month timepoint for those who reported lactation for 9 months or longer.[26] Another study documented persistent radial and tibial cortical and trabecular deficits versus baseline at a timepoint after breastfeeding (median of 3.6 years postpartum, range 0.9–5.4 years postpartum).[25]

The findings of site-specific BMD recovery patterns and persistent BMD and structural changes at distant postpartum timepoints should not necessarily be interpreted as having an adverse effect on skeletal structural competence or on fracture risk. Parity and lactation history have also been associated with larger bone size as well as greater bone strength in humans and in animal models.[16,29,30] A study of rats evaluated over 3 cycles of pregnancy/lactation documented lasting deficits in some aspects of trabecular structure, including trabecular number and connectivity density.

In contrast, cortical parameters improved over multiple reproductive cycles, with a net increase in cortical area and polar moment of inertia—suggesting that cortical bone adapts to increase load-bearing capacity and compensate for lasting trabecular changes.[2,16,17] Studies in rodent models also show that reproductive cycles lead to lasting microstructural skeletal changes that may be protective in the context of future menopausal bone loss.[31]

Data on BMD and structural changes observed during this dynamic time for bone should be placed in the context of the substantial evidence from multiple studies documenting no negative effect (and potential positive effects) of parity and lactation on fracture risk later in life.[32–37] In the Canadian Multicenter Osteoporosis Study, including 16 years of follow-up in over 3500 women (mean age 58 years), parity and lactation history showed no association with incident clinical or radiographic vertebral compression fractures.[32] In the Women's Health Initiative Observational Study, including over 93,000 postmenopausal women followed for a mean of 7.9 years, hip fracture incidence was not associated with parity, number of children breastfed, or total duration of breastfeeding.[33] Compared with never breastfeeding, a history of breastfeeding for greater than 1 month was associated with a *decreased* risk of hip fracture.[33] These large studies are relevant to expectations for long-term skeletal effects of pregnancy and lactation in healthy populations, but it remains possible that individuals with underlying disorders related to calcium or bone metabolism will have different overall trajectories and outcomes.

Clinical Implications of Pregnancy and Lactation Bone Physiology

One important clinical implication of these expected changes in bone mass around pregnancy and lactation is that BMD measured less than 12 months postpartum, particularly during lactation, is likely to be lower than that woman's baseline BMD and is likely to improve over time in the context of physiologic weaning/postweaning recovery. Reproductive history, including pregnancy and lactation history and timing details, should be obtained as part of interpretation of BMD results in premenopausal women.

An additional clinical implication is that, although skeletal demineralization and BMD decline is a physiologic and expected change associated with normal pregnancy and lactation, (1) some women may have bone or calcium metabolism disorders that alter the expected trajectory and (2) women with bone structure or quality deficits at baseline or with ongoing causes of bone fragility, may, rarely, be unable to tolerate these expected changes, and may sustain fractures during this time of skeletal stress and temporary structural vulnerability.

PREGNANCY AND LACTATION-ASSOCIATED OSTEOPOROSIS

PLO (sometimes abbreviated as PAO/LAO or PLAO) is a rare form of early onset osteoporosis characterized by fragility fractures that occur in the context of the expected bone mass and metabolism changes associated with pregnancy and lactation. The term PLO is often used to describe the clinical scenario of an initial, clinically severe, presentation with previously undiagnosed osteoporosis around pregnancy/lactation—and studies of PLO clinical characteristics, genetic characteristics, and treatment are often focused on this scenario. However, the term can also be used to describe any early onset osteoporosis, with known or unknown primary or secondary cause, which *includes* any fragility fractures sustained during pregnancy, during lactation, or shortly after reproductive events. Interpretation of reports on PLO clinical characteristics and treatment response should take into account the definition applied.

PLO was first described in the 1940 to 1950s[38,39] and has been clinically character-ized in several case reports[38,40–54] and a few case series, the largest including 24 to 177 women with PLO.[55–59] These case series document mean age at presentation of 27 to 39 years, often with multiple fractures (mean number of fractures 4 to 5 at pre-sentation).[55–57,59] The great majority are diagnosed with PLO during/after singleton pregnancy, but PLO during/after twin pregnancy has also been reported.[42,56] Women are often primiparous (67%–72%)[55–57,59] but may also be multiparous at the time of presentation/diagnosis. The majority of cases described (77%–93%) include vertebral fractures[55,56]; prominent symptoms include severe recurrent episodes of back pain and height loss. BMD before pregnancy is almost always unknown since there was no indication to previously measure it. At presentation, BMD by DXA is generally extremely low[1,54–56] with Z-scores often less than −3.0.

Some studies characterizing PLO have defined the condition based on vertebral fractures, while others include presentation with other types of fractures such as hip, sacral/pelvic, rib, and extremity fractures.[55–57] A condition sometimes termed "transient osteoporosis of the hip" (TOH) has been studied as a separate entity in the existing literature.[60,61] Since femoral marrow edema on MRI may also be inter-preted as representing evidence of femoral insufficiency/stress fracture,[59] distinct from avascular necrosis (AVN),[61,62] the previously identified TOH presentation may also be considered a hip insufficiency fracture presentation of PLO.[56,59,63]

Fracture timing in PLO is most commonly during lactation (in 79%–95%)[56,57] rather than during pregnancy—with pain onset at a mean of 2 ± 2 months postpartum.[56] Timing may differ by fracture type: a survey study of PLO documented that while ~90% of vertebral fractures presented during lactation, ~90% of hip fractures occurred during pregnancy.[56]

Case reports and case series highlight the disease severity of patients who come to medical attention and receive a diagnosis of PLO—and our interpretation of existing data on this condition may be affected by this bias. It is possible that some with fewer or less symptomatic vertebral fractures remain undiagnosed in the postpartum period and that some with fractures of sites other than the spine and hip are not identified as having PLO. Additionally, women with known osteogenesis imperfecta who sustain fractures during and after pregnancy are not generally categorized as having a PLO presentation.[64] Greater recognition of this condition and its presentation will broaden our understanding of clinical characteristics.

Most women identified with PLO are considered to have idiopathic osteoporosis (IOP)—and are reported to be otherwise healthy, with no known predisposing condition.[39,43,45,47,48,59] The great majority (~95%)[55,56] had not previously received a diagnosis of osteoporosis prior to the PLO presentation. Some studies have limited the PLO diagnosis to those with idiopathic PLO,[57,65] while other case reports, case se-ries, and treatment studies report potential secondary causes, including anorexia nerv-osa,[59,66,67] steroid exposure,[55,56,59] suppressive thyroid hormone therapy,[44] hyperthyroidism,[67] prolactinoma,[43] nephrolithiasis (which may be related to conditions associated with primary hypercalciuria),[56,63,68] celiac disease,[55,56] and heparin or low molecular weight heparin (LMWH) exposure.[49,54–56,59,61,67] In a survey study (n = 177), both heparin/LMWH exposure during pregnancy (reported by 14%) and celiac dis-ease (reported by 6%) were associated with more severe disease (more fractures)[56]; heparin/LMWH exposure was associated with earlier presentation (at mean of 1 ± 1 months postpartum vs 2 ± 2 months postpartum in those without exposure to hep-arins; $P = .001$).[56] It is possible that these factors alter the expected bone and calcium metabolism of pregnancy and lactation. Active celiac disease may be a cause of pre-existing bone fragility[69] and may also interfere with the process of adaptive calcium hyperabsorption expected during pregnancy. Heparins have been shown to decrease bone formation and increase bone resorption in animal models.[70–72] Treatment with heparins around pregnancy may interfere with bone remodeling adaptations during this time and/or may exacerbate underlying bone remodeling abnormalities. Because many of the earlier mentioned potential secondary causes are relatively common, and PLO presentation is quite rare and often severe, it is possible that some women with PLO have both primary/genetic osteoporosis and also secondary causes or disease modifiers that contribute to the presentation.

Genetic Characteristics of Pregnancy and Lactation-Associated Osteoporosis

The early onset, disease severity, lack of a known secondary cause in most, and reports of family history in approximately 50%[55,56] suggest a potential primary or genetic etiology of PLO. Reports document potentially disease-related variants in COL1A1 and COL1A2,[63,73] PLS3 (heterozygous),[68] LRP5 (heterozygous or compound heterozygous findings),[63,68,74,75] WNT1 (heterozygous),[63] ALPL (heterozygous),[63] and SLC34A3 (heterozygous).[63,68] In the largest PLO genetics study to date (n = 42), gene panel screening documenting heterozygous variants considered relevant to the condition in 50% and relevant variants in LRP5 or WNT1, which relate to the WNT signaling pathway, crucial for bone formation, in 26%.[63] The subgroup with relevant genetic variants had more severe disease, with higher number of fractures (4.8 ± 3.7 vs 1.8 ± 2.3; P = .02) among those wtih vertebral fractures,[63] but effects of potential genetic etiologies on prognosis of PLO remain unclear. It is notable that, although the most common genetic findings relate to bone formation pathways, findings to date suggest multiple potential disease mechanisms relating to abnormalities in bone formation, bone structure, and renal calcium handling.

Bone Structural Features of Pregnancy and Lactation-Associated Osteoporosis

Extremely low BMD by DXA, with spine T or Z score often less than −3.0, has been reported in PLO.[54–56] Consistent with the vertebral fracture presentation commonly noted in PLO, spine BMD is usually lower than hip BMD.[63,76] In Agarwal and colleagues 57 treatment-naïve women with PLO were compared to 2 control groups: treatment-naïve premenopausal women with IOP with fractures unrelated to pregnancy/lactation (non-PLO IOP; n = 47) and healthy nonosteoporotic premenopausal controls (n = 26), finding that women with PLO had a severe spine-predominant osteoporosis—with lower BMD than controls and those with IOP unrelated to pregnancy.[76,77] BMD was significantly lower at the spine and hip in PLO participants evaluated less than 12 months postpartum versus those evaluated at later timepoints, more distant from presentation and after expected postpartum BMD recovery.[76,77] In an assessment of vBMD, bone structure, and strength via central quantitative CT of the spine, the PLO group (n = 50) had significantly lower trabecular vBMD, vertebral integral BMD, and strength index in comparison to controls (n = 34).[76] Volumetric BMD, bone structure, and strength at the peripheral skeleton has been examined via HR-pQCT in several studies.[63,77,78] Scioscia and colleagues found that 7 PLO participants, studied 2 to 52 months postpartum, had lower total and trabecular density at the radius and lower trabecular number/higher trabecular separation at the radius and tibia in comparison to 8 healthy lactating women[79]; cortical density and thickness did not differ significantly between the groups. Butscheidt and colleagues[63] reported that, in comparison to age-specific and sex-specific normative data, 23 PLO women had lower vBMD and thickness for both the cortical and trabecular compartments, with no significant difference in trabecular number. In a study of 46 PLO participants,

Agarwal and colleagues also documented profound trabecular structural deficits versus controls and lower trabecular density and thickness in comparison to non-PLO IOP.[77]

Bone Remodeling Characteristics in Pregnancy and Lactation-Associated Osteoporosis

Tissue-level bone remodeling activity in PLO has been defined using transiliac crest bone biopsies after double tetracycline labeling. In a comparison of biopsy results between14 with PLO, 61 non-PLO IOP and 40 normal controls,[80] the PLO group had significantly lower mineral apposition rate than both non-PLO IOP and controls and significantly lower bone formation rate than non-PLO IOP. In this study, biopsies were assessed in PLO participants who were treatment naïve and greater than 12 months postpartum. Thus, findings are likely to reflect the baseline, inherent, bone remodeling status rather than postpartum changes—and suggest a predominantly low bone turnover phenotype in PLO. Future investigation will be needed to relate this tissue level finding to genetic findings, particularly given the evidence of genetic etiologies related to bone formation pathways in some.

This finding of a predominantly low bone turnover phenotype has several implications for treatment expectations in PLO. Since bone remodeling rate can be slow, bone-anabolic medications are expected to be more targeted for this condition than antiresorptive medications. However, low bone turnover also predicts less robust response to teriparatide in premenopausal IOP[81,82]—suggesting that some may have bone formation defects or osteoblast functional defects that create an environment that is less responsive to teriparatide. Further investigation is needed to determine response characteristics in PLO, for teriparatide as well as for new and emerging bone anabolic medications.

Evaluation and Initial Management After Presentation with Pregnancy and Lactation-Associated Osteoporosis

As with other presentations of early onset osteoporosis in adulthood, clinical evaluation should focus on a search for both primary and secondary etiologies of bone fragility.[1,83–85] Nonosteoporosis etiologies such as malignancy and osteomalacia should also be considered. When a secondary cause is identified, treatment of the underlying condition can be an important aspect of the management approach.

Evaluation should include an assessment of fracture status. In those with known or suspected vertebral fractures, this can include lumbar and thoracic spine imaging to quantify the number and severity of fractures both as a baseline for future comparison and as a potential predictor of future fracture risk.[57]

Pain management for acute and chronic symptoms and long-term rehabilitation are important aspects of care—but few guidelines exist to guide approaches for this rare condition.

Since bone density may decline with continued lactation, and bone recovery is expected to be aided by weaning and return of menses, options regarding cessation/limited duration of lactation are generally discussed as part of an initial management plan. Vitamin D should be supplemented to greater than 30 ng/mL to optimize calcium absorption. If there are no contraindications, calcium supplementation to achieve intake of 1 g/d can be recommended based on randomized trial evidence that calcium supplementation improves postweaning recovery in healthy women.[19]

Natural History and Prognosis of Pregnancy and Lactation-Associated Osteoporosis

Because PLO presents during the postpartum period, a very dynamic time for bone, expected bone mass changes during this time must be incorporated into understanding of prognosis. Two observational studies of PLO document BMD change in 5 to 8 untreated women with PLO.[65,67] BMD increased by an average of 7.5 ± 7.1% (adjusted analysis)[65] and 6.2 ± 4.8%,[67] on average, at the spine after 12 months of follow-up; there was substantial variability in BMD change observed. Studies of untreated women with PLO evaluated more than 12 months postpartum show that BMD remains quite low after the expected period of bone mass recovery, with an average spine Z score less than −2.0.[66,79] Several studies have documented prolonged pain and disability with variable trajectory of recovery in PLO.[57,86,87] Fracture risk appears to remain high after PLO diagnosis, with recurrent fractures in 20% to 39% in some reports.[54,58,88] In one study including 107 treated and untreated women with PLO, followed for a median of 6 years, 24% had additional fractures, 96% of these had vertebral fractures, and the number of fractures at diagnosis predicted subsequent risk.[57,58] Among 30 women with subsequent pregnancies, recurrent fractures were reported by 6 out of 30 (20%).[57,58] Another study reported recurrent fractures in 2 out of 7 women with subsequent pregnancy.[88] A study of women with TOH reported TOH recurrence in subsequent pregnancy in 2 out of 15 (13%).[61] In contrast, a report of 14 teriparatide-treated women with PLO who had subsequent pregnancies documented no fracture recurrence.[89]

Treatment of Pregnancy and Lactation-Associated Osteoporosis

Because the scenario identified as PLO is usually associated with multiple fractures affecting major sites and extremely low BMD at presentation, and because follow-up off therapy appears to be associated with ongoing fracture risk, treatment with medications aimed at improving bone quality is often recommended. It should be noted that cessation of lactation and effective contraception are both required to initiate medications for osteoporosis. Few clinical studies have assessed treatment effects in premenopausal women in general and in PLO specifically, and studies have been too small to draw conclusions regarding fracture risk reduction.

Most women with PLO are considered to have idiopathic or primary osteoporosis, thus the available data on treatment of adults with primary osteoporosis or IOP can be helpful to guide management for PLO. Several studies have documented BMD improvement in adults with osteogenesis imperfecta in the context of treatment with oral bisphosphonates, intravenous bisphosphonates, denosumab, and teriparatide.[90–94] Studies are generally too small to draw conclusions regarding fracture endpoints, do not specifically evaluate premenopausal female populations, and have not addressed treatment response in the postpartum setting. In premenopausal women with IOP, initiating treatment at least 12 months postpartum in those with pregnancy history, treatment with teriparatide over 24 months improved BMD by 13% at the spine and 5% at hip sites, on average, but response was variable with nonresponse in approximately 18%.[81,95] Treatment with sequential teriparatide and denosumab was associated with continued gains in areal BMD and vBMD.[96–98] In a study of 13 premenopausal women followed off additional therapy after teriparatide cessation for an average of 2 years, BMD declined by 4 ± 4% at the spine but remained stable at hip sites.[99] These data contribute to understanding of expectations for treatment response, particularly for idiopathic PLO, but do not address expectations for response to therapy initiated less than 12 months postpartum, during the time of physiologic postpartum bone mass changes.

No randomized trials have assessed treatment efficacy in newly diagnosed patients with PLO. Case reports and series document BMD improvement with several medications,[1] including bisphosphonates,[100] teriparatide,[43] denosumab,[101] and romosozumab[102]—but these studies do not report comparison to untreated controls. Two observational studies of teriparatide treatment in 19 to 27 postpartum patients with PLO have included small groups (n = 5–8) of untreated postpartum women with PLO[65,67]—allowing a comparison between treated and untreated postpartum BMD trajectory that is important for judging the effect of treatment during this dynamic time for the skeleton. In a study of 32 newly diagnosed women with idiopathic PLO and documented vertebral fractures, including approximately 20% previously treated with bisphosphonates for less than 6 months, Hong and colleagues[65] found that 12 month spine BMD increases were significantly larger in teriparatide-treated subjects (n = 27; +15.5 ± 6.6%, adjusted for age and baseline BMD) in comparison to untreated controls (+7.5 ± 7.1%, adjusted for age and baseline BMD; P = .02), with significant between groups differences seen at the total hip and femoral neck, as well. The BMD response to teriparatide varied widely, with spine BMD increase of +4.5% to +34.3%.[65] While baseline bone turnover markers did not relate to spine BMD response, there was a correlation (r = 0.4–0.5; P < .05) between spine BMD response and osteocalcin change at 3 and 6 months of treatment. It is not clear if prior bisphosphonate treatment could have contributed to the magnitude or variability of teriparatide response. Lampropoulou-Adamidou and colleagues[67] reported similar results in a study of 27 treatment-naïve women with PLO (some with secondary causes) and vertebral fractures, finding significant differences between the teriparatide treated (n = 19) and untreated (n = 8) groups for spine BMD change at 12 months (+20.9 ± 11.9 vs +6.2 ± 4.8; P < .001), but widely variable BMD change at the hip sites did not differ between treated and untreated groups. These studies document that teriparatide augments bone recovery postpartum in women with PLO and vertebral fractures in comparison to untreated (other than calcium/vitamin D) recovery, but response was quite variable and effects on fracture risk remain unknown.

One study has shown that, after teriparatide cessation, BMD gains are maintained without sequential antiresorptive treatment in women with idiopathic PLO.[89] This contrasts with the trajectory that was observed in women with IOP who lost bone, on average, after teriparatide cessation.[99] In a retrospective cohort study, Lee and colleagues compared 13 teriparatide-treated women with PLO who received various sequential antiresorptive treatments after teriparatide to 20 teriparatide-treated women with PLO who were followed off additional therapy after teriparatide completion. Over 3 years of follow-up, BMD increases were maintained and BMD change did not differ between groups at spine and hip sites.[89] This study excluded women with both known primary and secondary causes of osteoporosis. Thus, the findings are relevant to those with idiopathic PLO but may not be as predictive in situations where there is an active or ongoing secondary cause of bone loss.

Individual decisions regarding treatment options depend on many factors. Choices regarding initial treatment and sequential treatment may be influenced by disease severity, known genetic etiologies, presence or absence of known secondary causes of bone loss, and future pregnancy plans. Some may choose observation of postpartum BMD trajectory off therapy, while others may choose medical therapy. Teriparatide is the most studied initial therapy for PLO and has been shown to augment postpartum BMD recovery.[65,67] A course of teriparatide without sequential antiresorptive therapy is one option, particularly for women with idiopathic PLO or for those planning pregnancy in the short term. However, response to teriparatide is very variable in studies of PLO,[65] and studies of IOP also suggest that nonresponse or poor response is possible.[81,95] Close BMD follow-up may be helpful to assess early response to teriparatide treatment of PLO. Sequential antiresorptive therapy may be considered for those with more severe disease, inadequate teriparatide response, or ongoing causes of bone loss. Sequential treatment with teriparatide followed by denosumab leads to continued BMD and bone structural gains in premenopausal women with IOP.[96–98] Current guidelines recommend transition to alternative antiresorptive after denosumab cessation due to the risk of bone loss and fractures in this context, particularly in patients with vertebral fracture history.[103,104] In IOP, bone mass gains achieved with sequential teriparatide–denosumab were maintained with transition to bisphosphonate for 12 months after denosumab cessation.[105] Initial treatment with denosumab or bisphosphonates for PLO has been associated with BMD increase in case reports and case series[1]—but expectations for BMD trajectory with a denosumab–bisphosphonate sequence for PLO are unknown. Bisphosphonates have a long skeletal retention time and can cross the placenta, leading to potential concerns regarding safe use in women of childbearing potential. Issues relating to use of bisphosphonates before pregnancy have been previously reviewed.[19,83,85,106,107] Decisions regarding sequential therapy for osteoporosis in premenopausal women should consider risks related to treatment duration as well as plans for future pregnancy.

Many unanswered questions remain regarding PLO etiology, optimal treatment, and prognosis. Additional investigation is needed to elucidate genetic, metabolic, and structural mechanisms that lead to PLO—including factors that influence timing and severity of clinical presentation. Further therapeutic research is needed to determine whether mechanistic insights regarding PLO can guide tailored treatment approaches using current and emerging osteoporosis therapies. In parallel, long-term follow-up studies are needed to determine effects of treatment on future fracture risk.

CLINICS CARE POINTS

- Normal pregnancy and lactation are states of high calcium demand and are associated with substantial changes in bone metabolism and bone density.

- Multiple studies document no negative effect (and potential positive effects) of parity and lactation on fracture risk later in life.

- BMD measured less than 12 months postpartum, particularly during lactation, is likely to be lower than that woman's baseline BMD and is likely to improve over time in the context of physiologic weaning/postweaning recovery. Reproductive history, including pregnancy and lactation history and timing details, should be obtained as part of interpretation of BMD results in premenopausal women.

- PLO (sometimes abbreviated as PAO/LAO or PLAO) is a term used to describe an early onset osteoporosis presentation with fragility fractures that occur in the context of the bone mass and metabolism changes associated with pregnancy and lactation. The majority of cases identified as PLO include vertebral fracture(s); symptom onset is usually during lactation, rather than during pregnancy. Very low BMD by DXA and volumetric/structural bone deficits have been documented.

- As with other presentations of early onset osteoporosis in adulthood, clinical evaluation in PLO should focus on a search for both primary and secondary etiologies of bone fragility. Some with PLO have secondary causes of osteoporosis, some may have genetic etiologies/primary osteoporosis, some may have multiple potential etiologies/contributing factors, and many cases are considered idiopathic.

- Individual decisions regarding treatment options depend on many factors. Choices regarding initial treatment and sequential treatment may be influenced by disease severity, known genetic etiologies of bone fragility, presence or absence of known secondary causes of bone loss, and future pregnancy plans.
- Teriparatide is the most studied initial therapy for PLO and has been shown to augment postpartum BMD recovery. A course of teriparatide without sequential antiresorptive therapy is one option, particularly for women with idiopathic PLO or for those planning pregnancy in the short term.
- Response to teriparatide is variable in studies of PLO. Close BMD follow-up may be helpful to assess early response to teriparatide treatment for PLO.
- Sequential antiresorptive therapy may be considered for those with more severe disease, inadequate teriparatide response, or ongoing causes of bone loss.

DISCLOSURE

The author has received research funding from Amgen and Eli Lilly.

FUNDING

CUIMC research presented has been funded by the United States Food and Drug Administration (FDA) Orphan Products Clinical Trials Grants Program (R01 FD003902; R01 FD005114), and Natural History Studies Grants Program (R01 FD006007), the National Institutes of Health / National Institute of Arthritis and Musculoskeletal and Skin Diseases (R01 AR049896, K23 AR054127, R03 AR064016), Amgen, Eli Lilly, Thomas L. Kempner, Jr. and Katheryn C. Patterson and the Simon-Strauss Foundation.

REFERENCES

1. Hardcastle SA. Pregnancy and Lactation Associated Osteoporosis. Calcif Tissue Int 2022;110(5):531–45.
2. Kovacs CS. Maternal Mineral and Bone Metabolism During Pregnancy, Lactation, and Post-Weaning Recovery. Physiol Rev 2016;96(2):449–547.
3. Athonvarangkul D, Wysolmerski JJ. Crosstalk within a brain-breast-bone axis regulates mineral and skeletal metabolism during lactation. Front Physiol 2023;14:1121579.
4. Nakayama S, Yasui T, Suto M, et al. Differences in bone metabolism between singleton pregnancy and twin pregnancy. Bone 2011;49(3):513–9.
5. Naylor KE, Iqbal P, Fledelius C, et al. The effect of pregnancy on bone density and bone turnover. J Bone Miner Res 2000;15(1):129–37.
6. Black AJ, Topping J, Durham B, et al. A detailed assessment of alterations in bone turnover, calcium homeostasis, and bone density in normal pregnancy. J Bone Miner Res 2000;15(3):557–63.
7. Purdie DW, Aaron JE, Selby PL. Bone histology and mineral homeostasis in human pregnancy. Br J Obstet Gynaecol 1988;95(9):849–54.
8. Miyamoto T, Miyakoshi K, Sato Y, et al. Changes in bone metabolic profile associated with pregnancy or lactation. Sci Rep 2019;9(1):6787.
9. Sowers M, Eyre D, Hollis BW, et al. Biochemical markers of bone turnover in lactating and nonlactating postpartum women. J Clin Endocrinol Metab 1995; 80(7):2210–6.

10. Wysolmerski JJ. Osteocytes remove and replace perilacunar mineral during reproductive cycles. Bone 2013;54(2):230–6.

11. Bowman BM, Siska CC, Miller SC. Greatly increased cancellous bone formation with rapid improvements in bone structure in the rat maternal skeleton after lactation. J Bone Miner Res 2002;17(11):1954–60.

12. Ardeshirpour L, Dann P, Adams DJ, et al. Weaning triggers a decrease in receptor activator of nuclear factor-kappaB ligand expression, widespread osteoclast apoptosis, and rapid recovery of bone mass after lactation in mice. Endocrinology 2007;148(8):3875–86.

13. Karlsson MK, Ahlborg HG, Karlsson C. Maternity and bone mineral density. Acta Orthop 2005;76(1):2–13.

14. Moller UK, Vieth Streym S, Mosekilde L, et al. Changes in bone mineral density and body composition during pregnancy and postpartum. A controlled cohort study. Osteoporosis Int 2012;23(4):1213–23.

15. Sowers M, Crutchfield M, Jannausch M, et al. A prospective evaluation of bone mineral change in pregnancy. Obstet Gynecol 1991;77(6):841–5.

16. Liu XS, Wang L, de Bakker CMJ, et al. Mechanical Regulation of the Maternal Skeleton during Reproduction and Lactation. Curr Osteoporos Rep 2019; 17(6):375–86.

17. de Bakker CM, Altman-Singles AR, Li Y, et al. Adaptations in the Microarchitecture and Load Distribution of Maternal Cortical and Trabecular Bone in Response to Multiple Reproductive Cycles in Rats. J Bone Miner Res 2017; 32(5):1014–26.

18. M OB, Prentice A, Ward K. Pregnancy-Related Bone Mineral and Microarchitecture Changes in Women Aged 30 to 45 Years. J Bone Miner Res 2020;35(7): 1253–62.

19. Kalkwarf HJ, Specker BL, Bianchi DC, et al. The effect of calcium supplementation on bone density during lactation and after weaning. N Engl J Med 1997; 337(8):523–8.

20. Sowers M, Corton G, Shapiro B, et al. Changes in bone density with lactation. JAMA 1993;269(24):3130–5.

21. Karlsson C, Obrant KJ, Karlsson M. Pregnancy and lactation confer reversible bone loss in humans. Osteoporosis Int 2001;12(10):828–34.

22. Kolthoff N, Eiken P, Kristensen B, et al. Bone mineral changes during pregnancy and lactation: a longitudinal cohort study. Clin Sci 1998;94(4):405–12.

23. Lovelady CA, Bopp MJ, Colleran HL, et al. Effect of exercise training on loss of bone mineral density during lactation. Med Sci Sports Exerc 2009;41(10): 1902–7.

24. Li Y, de Bakker CMJ, Lai X, et al. Maternal bone adaptation to mechanical loading during pregnancy, lactation, and post-weaning recovery. Bone 2021; 151:116031.

25. Bjørnerem Å, Ghasem-Zadeh A, Wang X, et al. Irreversible deterioration of cortical and trabecular microstructure associated with breastfeeding. J Bone Miner Res 2017;32(4):681–7.

26. Brembeck P, Lorentzon M, Ohlsson C, et al. Changes in cortical volumetric bone mineral density and thickness, and trabecular thickness in lactating women postpartum. J Clin Endocrinol Metabol 2015;100(2):535–43.

27. Vajda EG, Bowman BM, Miller SC. Cancellous and cortical bone mechanical properties and tissue dynamics during pregnancy, lactation, and postlactation in the rat. Biol Reprod 2001;65(3):689–95.

28. Brembeck P, Lorentzon M, Ohlsson C, et al. Changes in cortical volumetric bone mineral density and thickness, and trabecular thickness in lactating women postpartum. J Clin Endocrinol Metab 2015;100(2):535–43.
29. Wiklund PK, Xu L, Wang Q, et al. Lactation is associated with greater maternal bone size and bone strength later in life. Osteoporosis Int 2012;23(7):1939–45.
30. Specker B, Binkley T. High parity is associated with increased bone size and strength. Osteoporosis Int 2005;16(12):1969–74.
31. de Bakker CM, Li Y, Zhao H, et al. Structural Adaptations in the Rat Tibia Bone Induced by Pregnancy and Lactation Confer Protective Effects Against Future Estrogen Deficiency. J Bone Miner Res 2018;33(12):2165–76.
32. Cooke-Hubley S, Gao Z, Mugford G, et al. Parity and lactation are not associated with incident fragility fractures or radiographic vertebral fractures over 16 years of follow-up: Canadian Multicentre Osteoporosis Study (CaMos). Arch Osteoporosis 2019;14(1):49.
33. Crandall CJ, Liu J, Cauley J, et al. Associations of Parity, Breastfeeding, and Fractures in the Women's Health Observational Study. Obstet Gynecol 2017;130(1):171–80.
34. Alderman BW, Weiss NS, Daling JR, et al. Reproductive history and postmenopausal risk of hip and forearm fracture. Am J Epidemiol 1986;124(2):262–7.
35. Cummings SR, Nevitt MC, Browner WS, et al. Risk factors for hip fracture in white women. Study of Osteoporotic Fractures Research Group. N Engl J Med 1995;332(12):767–73.
36. Michaelsson K, Baron JA, Farahmand BY, et al. Influence of parity and lactation on hip fracture risk. Am J Epidemiol 2001;153(12):1166–72.
37. Karlsson MK, Ahlborg HG, Karlsson C. Female reproductive history and the skeleton-a review. BJOG 2005;112(7):851–6.
38. Nordin BE, Roper A. Post-pregnancy osteoporosis; a syndrome? Lancet 1955;268(6861):431–4.
39. Kovacs CS, Ralston SH. Presentation and management of osteoporosis presenting in association with pregnancy or lactation. Osteoporosis Int 2015;26(9):2223–41.
40. Vujasinovic-Stupar N, Pejnovic N, Markovic L, et al. Pregnancy-associated spinal osteoporosis treated with bisphosphonates: long-term follow-up of maternal and infants outcome. Rheumatol Int 2012;32(3):819–23.
41. Sarikaya S, Ozdolap S, Acikgoz G, et al. Pregnancy-associated osteoporosis with vertebral fractures and scoliosis. Joint Bone Spine : Rev Rhum 2004;71(1):84–5.
42. Grizzo FM, da Silva Martins J, Pinheiro MM, et al. Pregnancy and Lactation-Associated Osteoporosis: Bone Histomorphometric Analysis and Response to Treatment with Zoledronic Acid. Calcif Tissue Int 2015;97(4):421–5.
43. Choe EY, Song JE, Park KH, et al. Effect of teriparatide on pregnancy and lactation-associated osteoporosis with multiple vertebral fractures. J Bone Miner Metabol 2012;30(5):596–601.
44. Lampropoulou-Adamidou K, Trovas G, Stathopoulos IP, et al. Case report: Teriparatide treatment in a case of severe pregnancy -and lactation- associated osteoporosis. Hormones (Basel) 2012;11(4):495–500.
45. Hellmeyer L, Boekhoff J, Hadji P. Treatment with teriparatide in a patient with pregnancy-associated osteoporosis. Gynecol Endocrinol 2010;26(10):725–8.
46. Blanch J, Pacifici R, Chines A. Pregnancy-associated osteoporosis: report of two cases with long-term bone density follow-up. Br J Rheumatol 1994;33(3):269–72.

47. Iwamoto J, Sato Y, Uzawa M, et al. Five-year follow-up of a woman with pregnancy and lactation-associated osteoporosis and vertebral fractures. Therapeut Clin Risk Manag 2012;8:195–9.

48. Nakamura Y, Kamimura M, Ikegami S, et al. A case series of pregnancy- and lactation-associated osteoporosis and a review of the literature. Therapeut Clin Risk Manag 2015;11:1361–5.

49. Ozdemir D, Tam AA, Dirikoc A, et al. Postpartum osteoporosis and vertebral fractures in two patients treated with enoxaparin during pregnancy. Osteoporosis Int 2015;26(1):415–8.

50. Yamamoto N, Takahashi HE, Tanizawa T, et al. Bone mineral density and bone histomorphometric assessments of postpregnancy osteoporosis: a report of five patients. Calcif Tissue Int 1994;54(1):20–5.

51. Phillips AJ, Ostlere SJ, Smith R. Pregnancy-associated osteoporosis: does the skeleton recover? Osteoporosis Int 2000;11(5):449–54.

52. Ozturk C, Atamaz FC, Akkurt H, et al. Pregnancy-associated osteoporosis presenting severe vertebral fractures. J Obstet Gynaecol Res 2014;40(1):288–92.

53. Bonacker J, Janousek M, Krober M. Pregnancy-associated osteoporosis with eight fractures in the vertebral column treated with kyphoplasty and bracing: a case report. Arch Orthop Trauma Surg 2014;134(2):173–9.

54. Hardcastle SA, Yahya F, Bhalla AK. Pregnancy-associated osteoporosis: a UK case series and literature review. Osteoporosis Int 2019;30(5):939–48.

55. Dunne F, Walters B, Marshall T, et al. Pregnancy associated osteoporosis. Clin Endocrinol 1993;39(4):487–90.

56. Kondapalli AV, Kamanda-Kosseh M, Williams JM, et al. Clinical characteristics of pregnancy and lactation associated osteoporosis: An online survey study. Osteoporosis Int 2023;34(8):1477–89.

57. Kyvernitakis I, Reuter TC, Hellmeyer L, et al. Subsequent fracture risk of women with pregnancy and lactation-associated osteoporosis after a median of 6 years of follow-up. Osteoporosis Int 2018;29(1):135–42.

58. Kyvernitakis I, Reuter TC, Hellmeyer L, et al. Correction to: Subsequent fracture risk of women with pregnancy and lactation-associated osteoporosis after a median of 6 years of follow-up. Osteoporosis Int 2023;34(12):2143–4.

59. Smith R, Athanasou NA, Ostlere SJ, et al. Pregnancy-associated osteoporosis. QJM : monthly journal of the Association of Physicians 1995;88(12):865–78.

60. Hadji P, Boekhoff J, Hahn M, et al. Pregnancy-associated transient osteoporosis of the hip: results of a case-control study. Arch Osteoporos 2017;12(1):11.

61. Toussia-Cohen S, Eshed I, Segal O, et al. Transient osteoporosis of the hip in pregnancy - a case series. J Matern Fetal Neonatal Med 2023;36(1):2175659.

62. Malizos KN, Zibis AH, Dailiana Z, et al. MR imaging findings in transient osteoporosis of the hip. Eur J Radiol 2004;50(3):238–44.

63. Butscheidt S, Tsourdi E, Rolvien T, et al. Relevant genetic variants are common in women with pregnancy and lactation-associated osteoporosis (PLO) and predispose to more severe clinical manifestations. Bone 2021;147:115911.

64. Koumakis E, Cormier-Daire V, Dellal A, et al. Osteogenesis Imperfecta: characterization of fractures during pregnancy and post-partum. Orphanet J Rare Dis 2022;17(1):22.

65. Hong N, Kim JE, Lee SJ, et al. Changes in bone mineral density and bone turnover markers during treatment with teriparatide in pregnancy- and lactation-associated osteoporosis. Clin Endocrinol 2018;88(5):652–8.

66. Kasahara K, Kita N, Kawasaki T, et al. Bilateral femoral neck fractures resulting from pregnancy-associated osteoporosis showed bone marrow edema on magnetic resonance imaging. J Obstet Gynaecol Res 2017;43(6):1067–70.

67. Lampropoulou-Adamidou K, Trovas G, Triantafyllopoulos IK, et al. Teriparatide Treatment in Patients with Pregnancy- and Lactation-Associated Osteoporosis. Calcif Tissue Int 2021;109(5):554–62.

68. Cohen A, Hostyk J, Baugh EH, et al. Whole exome sequencing reveals potentially pathogenic variants in a small subset of premenopausal women with idiopathic osteoporosis. Bone 2022;154:116253.

69. Leffler DA, Green PH, Fasano A. Extraintestinal manifestations of coeliac disease. Nat Rev Gastroenterol Hepatol 2015;12(10):561–71.

70. Irie A, Takami M, Kubo H, et al. Heparin enhances osteoclastic bone resorption by inhibiting osteoprotegerin activity. Bone 2007;41(2):165–74.

71. Muir JM, Andrew M, Hirsh J, et al. Histomorphometric analysis of the effects of standard heparin on trabecular bone in vivo. Blood 1996;88(4):1314–20.

72. Shaughnessy SG, Young E, Deschamps P, et al. The effects of low molecular weight and standard heparin on calcium loss from fetal rat calvaria. Blood 1995;86(4):1368–73.

73. Pabinger C, Heu C, Frohner A, et al. Pregnancy- and lactation-associated transient osteoporosis of both hips in a 32 year old patient with osteogenesis imperfecta. Bone 2012;51(1):142–4.

74. Campos-Obando N, Oei L, Hoefsloot LH, et al. Osteoporotic vertebral fractures during pregnancy: be aware of a potential underlying genetic cause. J Clin Endocrinol Metab 2014;99(4):1107–11.

75. Cook FJ, Mumm S, Whyte MP, et al. Pregnancy-associated osteoporosis with a heterozygous deactivating LDL receptor-related protein 5 (LRP5) mutation and a homozygous methylenetetrahydrofolate reductase (MTHFR) polymorphism. J Bone Miner Res 2014;29(4):922–8.

76. Agarwal S, Lang T, Kamanda-Kosseh M, et al. Women with pregnancy and lactation associated osteoporosis (PLO) have substantial volumetric BMD deficits at the spine by central QCT. Vancouver, BC: Paper presented at: American Society for Bone and Mineral Research Annual Meeting; 2023.

77. Agarwal S, El-Najjar D, Kondapalli AV, et al. HRpQCT reveals marked trabecular and cortical structural deficits in women with pregnancy and lactation associated osteoporosis (PLO) - oral presentation. Austin, TX: Paper presented at: American Society for Bone and Mineral Research Annual Meeting; 2022.

78. Scioscia MF, Vidal M, Sarli M, et al. Severe Bone Microarchitecture Impairment in Women With Pregnancy and Lactation-Associated Osteoporosis. J Endocr Soc 2021;5(5):bvab031.

79. Scioscia MF, Vidal M, Sarli M, et al. Severe Bone Microarchitecture Impairment in Women With Pregnancy and Lactation-Associated Osteoporosis. Journal of the Endocrine Society 2021;5(5):bvab031.

80. Cohen A, Kamanda-Kosseh M, Dempster DW, et al. Women With Pregnancy and Lactation-Associated Osteoporosis (PLO) Have Low Bone Remodeling Rates at the Tissue Level. J Bone Miner Res 2019;34(9):1552–61.

81. Cohen A, Stein EM, Recker RR, et al. Teriparatide for idiopathic osteoporosis in premenopausal women: a pilot study. J Clin Endocrinol Metab 2013;98(5):1971–81.

82. Goetz TG, Nair N, Shiau S, et al. In premenopausal women with idiopathic osteoporosis, lower bone formation rate is associated with higher body fat and higher IGF-1. Osteoporosis Int 2022;3:659–72.

83. Becker C.B. and Cohen A., Evaluation and treatment of premenopasual osteo-porosis, In: UpToDate, Rosen C.J., Editor. Wolters Kluwer. Available at: https://www.uptodate.com/contents/evaluation-and-treatment-of-premenopausal-osteoporosis. (Accessed June 13, 2024).

84. Pepe J, Body JJ, Hadji P, et al. Osteoporosis in Premenopausal Women: A Clinical Narrative Review by the ECTS and the IOF. J Clin Endocrinol Metab 2020; 105(8):dgaa306.

85. Herath M, Cohen A, Ebeling PR, et al. Dilemmas in the Management of Osteo-porosis in Younger Adults. JBMR Plus 2022;6(1):e10594.

86. Gehlen M, Lazarescu AD, Hinz C, et al. Long-term outcome of patients with pregnancy and lactation-associated osteoporosis (PLO) with a particular focus on quality of life. Clin Rheumatol 2019;38(12):3575–83.

87. Peltz-Sinvani N, Raz HM, Klein P, et al. Pregnancy- and lactation-induced oste-oporosis: a social-media-based survey. BMC Pregnancy Childbirth 2023; 23(1):311.

88. Laroche M, Talibart M, Cormier C, et al. Pregnancy-related fractures: a retro-spective study of a French cohort of 52 patients and review of the literature. Osteoporosis Int 2017;28(11):3135–42.

89. Lee S, Hong N, Kim KJ, et al. Bone Density After Teriparatide Discontinuation With or Without Antiresorptive Therapy in Pregnancy- and Lactation-Associated Osteoporosis. Calcif Tissue Int 2021;109(5):544–53.

90. Liu W, Lee B, Nagamani SCS, et al. Approach to the Patient: Pharmacological Therapies for Fracture Risk Reduction in Adults With Osteogenesis Imperfecta. J Clin Endocrinol Metab 2023;108(7):1787–96.

91. Lin X, Hu J, Zhou B, et al. Efficacy and safety of denosumab vs zoledronic acid in OI adults: a prospective, open-label, randomized study. J Clin Endocrinol Metab 2024;109(7):1873–82.

92. Leali PT, Balsano M, Maestretti G, et al. Efficacy of teriparatide vs neridronate in adults with osteogenesis imperfecta type I: a prospective randomized interna-tional clinical study. Clin Cases Miner Bone Metab 2017;14(2):153–6.

93. Orwoll ES, Shapiro J, Veith S, et al. Evaluation of teriparatide treatment in adults with osteogenesis imperfecta. J Clin Invest 2014;124(2):491–8.

94. Dwan K, Phillipi CA, Steiner RD, et al. Bisphosphonate therapy for osteogenesis imperfecta. Cochrane Database Syst Rev 2016;10(10):CD005088.

95. Cohen A, Shiau S, Nair N, et al. Effect of Teriparatide on Bone Remodeling and Density in Premenopausal Idiopathic Osteoporosis: A Phase II Trial. J Clin Endo-crinol Metab 2020;105(10):e3540–56.

96. Agarwal S, Shane E, Lang T, et al. Spine volumetric BMD and strength in pre-menopausal idiopathic osteoporosis: Effect of teriparatide followed by denosu-mab. J Clin Endocrinol Metab 2022;107(7):e2690–701.

97. Agarwal S, Shiau S, Kamanda-Kosseh M, et al. Teriparatide Followed by Deno-sumab in Premenopausal Idiopathic Osteoporosis: Bone Microstructure and Strength by HR-pQCT. J Bone Miner Res 2023;38(1):35–47.

98. Shane E, Shiau S, Recker RR, et al. Denosumab after teriparatide in premeno-pausal women with idiopathic osteoporosis. J Clin Endocrinol Metab 2021; 107(4):e1528–40.

99. Cohen A, Kamanda-Kosseh M, Recker RR, et al. Bone Density after Teriparatide Discontinuation in Premenopausal Idiopathic Osteoporosis. J Clin Endocrinol Metab 2015;100(11):4208–14.

100. O'Sullivan SM, Grey AB, Singh R, et al. Bisphosphonates in pregnancy and lactation-associated osteoporosis. Osteoporosis Int 2006;17(7):1008–12.

101. Stumpf U, Kraus M, Hadji P. Influence of denosumab on bone mineral density in a severe case of pregnancy-associated osteoporosis. Osteoporosis Int 2021; 32(11):2383–7.

102. Kaneuchi Y, Iwabuchi M, Hakozaki M, et al. Pregnancy and Lactation-Associated Osteoporosis Successfully Treated with Romosozumab: A Case Report. Medicina (Kaunas) 2022;59(1):19.

103. Tsourdi E, Langdahl B, Cohen-Solal M, et al. Discontinuation of Denosumab therapy for osteoporosis: A systematic review and position statement by ECTS. Bone 2017;105:11–7.

104. Cummings SR, Ferrari S, Eastell R, et al. Vertebral Fractures After Discontinuation of Denosumab: A Post Hoc Analysis of the Randomized Placebo-Controlled FREEDOM Trial and Its Extension. J Bone Miner Res 2018;33(2):190–8.

105. Kamanda-Kosseh M, Shiau S, Agarwal S. et al. Bisphosphonates Maintain BMD after sequential teriparatide and denosumab in premenopausal women with idiopathic osteoporosis paper presented at: American Society for Bone and Mineral Research Annual Meeting, Vancouver, BC, Canada, October 2023.

106. Buckley L, Guyatt G, Fink HA, et al. 2017 American College of Rheumatology Guideline for the Prevention and Treatment of Glucocorticoid-Induced Osteoporosis. Arthritis Rheumatol 2017;69(8):1521–37.

107. Chakrabarti K, McCune WJ. Glucocorticoid-induced osteoporosis in premenopausal women: management for the rheumatologist. Curr Opin Rheumatol 2023;35(3):161–9.

Reproductive Considerations in the Transgender and Gender Diverse Population: A Review

Michele B. Glodowski, MD[a],*, Carlos M. Parra, MD[b], Madeline K. Xin, BA[c], Mary Elizabeth Fino, MD[b]

KEYWORDS

- Transgender • Transgender and gender diverse (TGD)
- Gender-affirming hormone therapy (GAHT) • Fertility • Fertility preservation
- Cryopreservation • Contraception • Adolescents

KEY POINTS

- Medically necessary gender-affirming hormone therapy and gender-affirming surgeries have a negative impact on reproductive potential, and all transgender and gender diverse individuals should be counseled regarding fertility prior to initiating gender-affirming treatments.
- Options for fertility preservation for patients who have undergone puberty include mature oocyte, embryo, and sperm cryopreservation.
- In prepubertal individuals assigned female sex at birth, ovarian tissue cryopreservation may be considered. In prepubertal individuals assigned male at birth, testicular tissue cryopreservation remains experimental only.
- This review aims to summarize the effects of gender-affirming hormone therapy on reproductive potential and discuss current and future options for fertility preservation in both adolescents and adults.

INTRODUCTION

It is estimated that over 1.6 million adults and adolescents identify as transgender or gender diverse in the United States, representing 0.6% of the population.[1] Extrapolating similar data globally, this number is 25 million people worldwide.[2] Many of these

[a] Division of Endocrinology, Diabetes and Metabolism, Department of Medicine, New York University Langone Health, 111 Broadway, 2nd Floor, New York, NY 10006, USA; [b] Division of Reproductive Endocrinology and Infertility, Department of Obstetrics & Gynecology, New York University Langone Prelude Fertility Center, 159 East 53rd Street, 3rd Floor, New York, NY 10022, USA; [c] NYU Grossman School of Medicine, 550 First Avenue, New York, NY 10016, USA
* Corresponding author. 111 Broadway, 2nd Floor, New York, NY 10006.
E-mail address: Michele.Glodowski@nyulangone.org

Endocrinol Metab Clin N Am 53 (2024) 471–482
https://doi.org/10.1016/j.ecl.2024.05.008
0889-8529/24/Published by Elsevier Inc.

individuals will be considering treatment with gender-affirming hormone therapy (GAHT) and/or gender-affirming surgery (GAS) during their reproductive lifespan, and several studies have demonstrated a desire for fertility among transgender and gender diverse (TGD) individuals. In a study by Wierckx and colleagues, more than half of the participants (54%) had a desire to have children.[3] In a study examining attitudes toward fertility among adolescents (median age 16 years), 35% were interested in biological parenthood.[4]

GAHT can include (but is not limited to) estrogens, antiandrogens (spironolactone, cyproterone acetate [CPA] where available), gonadotropin-releasing hormone agonists (GnRHas), and testosterone, often with the goal of bringing sex hormone levels into the physiologic range of the affirmed gender and allowing for changes to secondary sex characteristics. This helps to better align a person's physical appearance with their gender identity. While these treatments are an essential component of gender-affirming care, they have a negative impact on fertility.[5] Despite this, and despite a demonstrated interest in parenthood as abovementioned, rates of fertility preservation (FP) are low. In a recent study from Israel of 188 subjects, 67% of transgender women and 62% of transgender men reported wishing to parent a child; however, only 40% of transgender women and only 5.8% of transgender men reported completing FP.[6] Lower rates of FP were reported in a study from Germany in which 76% of transgender women and 77% of transgender men indicated that they had at least thought about FP; however, only 9.6% of transgender women and 3.1% of transgender men had completed FP.[7] Other studies similarly have demonstrated low rates of FP among TGD adolescents.[8,9]

While some studies report a decreased importance to being genetically related to offspring among reasons expressed for not pursuing FP,[10] other barriers reported include cost/lack of insurance coverage, need to delay GAHT, and fear of worsening of gender dysphoria with fertility treatments. Some studies also report concerns regarding the attitude of medical staff or being discriminated against as a TGD parent.[6,10,11]

Both the World Professional Association for Transgender Health (WPATH) and the American Society for Reproductive Medicine (ASRM) recommend that patients receiving gender-affirming treatments are counseled on the effects of GAHT and GAS on fertility as well as options for FP.[12,13] Counseling should be provided at each stage of transition, including before medical and surgical transition and before pubertal suppression in adolescents. This review aims to summarize the effects of GAHT on reproductive potential and discuss current and future options for FP in both adolescents and adults. It also discusses contraception and family planning as an important part of comprehensive reproductive health. **Table 1** summarizes the common terminology used in the literature and necessary terms for providing gender-inclusive care.

EFFECTS OF HORMONE THERAPY ON FERTILITY IN TRANSGENDER AND GENDER DIVERSE PEOPLE ASSIGNED MALE AT BIRTH

Estrogen—given orally, parenterally, or transdermally in the form of estradiol—is a central part of a feminizing hormone therapy regimen. Estrogen therapy alone at recommended doses does not reliably suppress testosterone to usual targets. Therefore, antiandrogens are frequently combined with estrogen. These may include GnRHa, spironolactone, or CPA depending on preference, although CPA is not currently available in the United States.[13]

Treatment with estrogen has been shown to decrease sperm production and cause testicular atrophy.[13–17] Histopathologic studies of the testes in transgender women

Table 1
Common terminology

	Definition
Cisgender	Someone whose current gender identity corresponds to their sex assigned at birth.
Gender	A broad social concept that can include gender identity, gender expression, and/or social gender role.
Gender affirmation	Recognition or affirmation of an individual's gender identity through social, psychological, medical, and/or legal contexts.
Gender-affirming surgery	Any surgery with the primary goal of altering primary and/or secondary sex characteristics to affirm an individual's gender identity.
Gender dysphoria	In common language, the experience of distress due to a difference between an individual's gender identity and the gender identity associated with their sex assigned at birth. Also, a diagnostic term in the diagnostic and statistical manual of mental disorders (DSM-5) denoting an incongruence between the sex assigned at birth and experienced gender, accompanied by distress.
Gender expression	How an individual expresses gender in their life, such as through appearance and/or behavior.
Gender identity	An individual's internal sense of their own gender.
Sex assigned at birth	An individual's status as male, female, or intersex based on physical characteristics. Sex is typically assigned at birth based on appearance of external genitalia.
Transfeminine	Someone who was assigned male at birth and has a gender identity that is more feminine than masculine.
Transgender or gender diverse	Broad terms used to describe individuals whose gender identity and/or gender expression differ from that expected of their sex assigned at birth. May include those who identify as nonbinary, gender nonconforming, and others who do not identify as cisgender.
Transition	The process of changing from the gender expression associated with sex assigned at birth to another gender expression that better fits an individual's gender identity.
Trans man	Someone who identities as a man and who was assigned female at birth.
Transmasculine	Someone who was assigned female at birth and has a gender identity that is more masculine than feminine.
Trans woman	Someone who identities as a woman and who was assigned male at birth.

Adapted from Coleman E, Radix AE, Bouman WP, et al. Standards of Care for the Health of Transgender and Gender Diverse People, Version 8. Int J Transgend Health. 2022;23(Suppl 1):S1-S259. Published 2022 Sep 6.

after orchiectomy show variable and conflicting results. The largest study by Jindarak and colleagues retrospectively studied 173 orchiectomy specimens after long-term treatment with GAHT and found normal spermatogenesis in 11%, with the remainder showing maturation arrest (36.4%), hypospermatogenesis (26%), Sertoli cell-only syndrome (20.2%), and seminiferous tubule hyalinization (6.4%).[14] Other studies have reported normal spermatogenesis in as low as 4% of specimens.[15] Still, Vereecke and colleagues found that complete spermatogenesis could not be found in any of their 97 participants at gonadectomy after treatment with CPA plus estrogen.[18] Furthermore, studies have failed to demonstrate a specific duration of treatment necessary to have a negative impact on fertility.[15,19] Limited case studies exist that reinforce the theoretic inverse dose–response relationship between estrogen and spermatogenesis,[20] and different combinations of estrogen and antiandrogens may lead to different levels of fertility impairment.[21]

Reversibility of fertility impairment upon cessation of hormone therapy may be possible but data are limited. Studies have shown wide variations in outcomes, with full restoration of spermatogenesis seen as early as 6 weeks or as late as 17 months following discontinuation of therapy.[22–24] For some patients, discontinuing all forms of hormonal therapy for such an extended time may not be an option, and so functional and achievable return of fertility remains an open-ended question.

EFFECTS OF HORMONE THERAPY ON FERTILITY IN TRANSGENDER AND GENDER DIVERSE PEOPLE ASSIGNED FEMALE AT BIRTH

GAHT for TGD individuals assigned female at birth includes testosterone. There is much variability in dosing depending on the individual goals of each patient, but typical testosterone targets are in the mid-normal physiologic range of cismen.[25] Testosterone therapy commonly leads to menstrual irregularities or amenorrhea due to suppressed ovulatory function within the first 6 to 12 months of treatment.[5,26] However, it is important to note that ovulation may still occur, and long-term treatment with testosterone alone is not an adequate form of contraception, with pregnancies reported in patients with amenorrhea on testosterone.[27]

Although it was once suspected that treatment with testosterone would induce polycystic ovarian morphology (PCOM) in trans men, studies show conflicting results. A study using 3D transvaginal ultrasound to evaluate for PCOM (defined as an antral follicle count of 12 or more in any ovary) found no difference between the transmasculine group on testosterone and the cisgender control group.[28] Histopathologic studies of the ovaries of transmasculine patients on testosterone after oophorectomy have shown greater numbers of atretic follicles but otherwise normal cortical follicle distribution, and while changes to the ovarian cortex as well as ovarian stromal hyperplasia and stromal luteinization were reported, evidence of complete PCOM was not.[29,30] In terms of long-term testosterone treatment's impact to the endometrium, studies have demonstrated both atrophy and proliferative endometrium, even in amenorrheic patients.[26,31,32]

Upon discontinuation of testosterone therapy, patients typically experience the resumption of regular menstrual cycles and ovulatory function within 6 months.[27] Retrospective data have shown no difference between ovarian stimulation outcomes in TGD men previously on hormone therapy and cisgender women,[33–35] and successful oocyte and embryo cryopreservation, pregnancy, and live births have all been reported after cessation of testosterone therapy.[34,36]

While overall data are promising, the effect of long-term androgen therapy on fertility is still somewhat unclear[37] and more prospective and long-term studies are needed.

EFFECTS OF GONADOTROPIN-RELEASING HORMONE AGONISTS ON FERTILITY IN TRANSGENDER AND GENDER DIVERSE ADOLESCENTS

TGD youth may be eligible for treatment with GnRHa once they reach at minimum Tanner stage 2 of puberty.[13] GnRHas exert their effect by disrupting the normally pulsatile GnRH signal from the hypothalamus to the pituitary. After a brief peak of follicle-stimulating hormone (FSH) and luteinizing hormone (LH) production, there is suppression of FSH, LH, and downstream hormones, typically by 4 weeks.[38] Such agents are used to "pause" puberty so that youth may more fully explore their gender identity and to delay the development of unwanted secondary sex characteristics.[39] GnRHas inhibit spermatogenesis and oocyte maturation, although when evaluating the use of GnRHa in precocious puberty, this effect is generally thought of as reversible once therapy is stopped.[40,41]

FERTILITY PRESERVATION

Most TGD individuals initiate gender-affirming care in their 20s at peak reproductive years when alleviating gender dysphoria is the main priority.[42] However, as previously mentioned, more than half of TGD individuals express a desire for future children, but only a minority pursues FP due to a variety of reasons including lack of counseling. Major organizations (such as ASRM and WPATH) strongly recommend that all TGD individuals receive counseling prior to initiating GAHT and/or GAS to discuss reproductive potential after transitioning and strategize for future family building if desired. Existing options for future reproduction include gonadal tissue cryopreservation (for prepubertal individuals), gametes or embryo cryopreservation (for postpubertal individuals), third party reproduction (such as donor sperm/mature oocytes and gestational carrier), and adoption. In this section, the focus will be on FP options for future genetically related children, which are summarized in **Table 2**.

OPTIONS FOR FERTILITY PRESERVATION IN TRANSGENDER AND GENDER DIVERSE PEOPLE ASSIGNED FEMALE AT BIRTH

For prepubertal transmasculine individuals starting pubertal blockers (GnRHa) followed by masculinizing hormones (testosterone), ovarian tissue cryopreservation prior to initiation of GnRHa is the most ideal FP option given the risk of reproductive function loss. Cryopreservation refers to the storage of cells or tissues at subzero temperatures to halt biological activity. In the context of patients with cancer at risk for gonadal injury, the ASRM removed the experimental label on ovarian tissue cryopreservation in 2019 and deemed it acceptable if hormonal preparation was not possible.[43] Hormonal preparation or controlled ovarian stimulation is needed for mature oocyte retrieval which may not be an option for patients required to start cancer-directed treatment within a short timeframe or TGD individuals who are prepubertal with an immature hypothalamic–pituitary–ovarian (HPO) axis. The process of ovarian tissue cryopreservation involves a surgical procedure by which ovarian cortical tissue is obtained via partial or complete oophorectomy performed laparoscopically or through laparotomy. The ovarian tissue is transported to the embryology laboratory for cryopreservation. When the patient is ready to procreate, the ovarian tissue is thawed and transplanted typically to its native anatomic site in the pelvis. This transplanted ovarian tissue is shown to regain function within 60 to 240 days and has resulted in more than 100 reported human live births.[43] Unfortunately, for individuals who wish to avoid future ovarian tissue transplantation, the most ideal FP option is mature oocyte cryopreservation for which a postpubertal functioning HPO axis is needed. While controlled ovarian stimulation for oocyte retrieval in prepubertal individuals on puberty blockers has been reported, there is a complete lack of outcome data, thus making it impractical.[44,45] The ability to retrieve immature oocytes from ovarian tissue and induce their in vitro maturation to mature oocytes for cryopreservation or fertilization remains experimental with only live births shown in animal models.[46]

For postpubertal transmasculine individuals starting masculinizing hormones (testosterone), the downregulation of the HPO axis leads to ovarian suppression and amenorrhea in uterine-retaining individuals. Although menses will return within 6 months for about 80% of transmasculine individuals after stopping testosterone,[27] the resumption of reproductive function is not guaranteed and, thus, mature oocyte

Table 2
Fertility preservation options for transgender and gender diverse individuals

	Prepubertal	Postpubertal
TGD individuals assigned female at birth	Ovarian tissue cryopreservation • Approved in all ages but only option if prepubertal • Ovarian cortical tissue obtained surgically without hormonal preparation • Requires thaw and transplantation for use in the future • Limited number of live births reported in humans	Mature oocyte cryopreservation • Only possible if postpubertal • Controlled ovarian stimulation to facilitate multifollicular ovarian growth followed by oocyte aspiration procedure • Requires thaw and in vitro fertilization for embryo creation in the future Embryo cryopreservation • Same as the above except immediate in vitro fertilization of fresh mature oocytes • Sperm source required from sexually intimate partner or donor (anonymous or known) • Requires thaw and transfer to uterine-retaining individuals (self, partner, or gestational carrier) in the future

TGD individuals assigned male at birth	Testicular tissue cryopreservation
	• Experimental in all ages but primarily in prepubertal
	• Testicular tissue obtained surgically
	• Successful outcomes in animal models but no live births reported in humans
		Sperm cryopreservation
		• Only possible if postpubertal
		• Sperm sample usually obtained via masturbation
		  ○ Assistive ejaculatory methods: electroejaculation, penile vibratory stimulation
		  ○ Nonejaculatory methods: testicular or epididymal sperm aspiration
		• Requires thaw to be used for artificial insemination or in vitro fertilization in the future

or embryo cryopreservation prior to masculinizing hormone therapy is the most ideal FP option. The process of mature oocyte cryopreservation (or egg freezing) requires patients to be a Tanner stage 4 or greater and entails 10 to 12 days of hormonal preparation followed by a surgical procedure. During this time, individuals undergo controlled ovarian stimulation via daily injectable gonadotropins (FSH or LH) to stimulate ovarian follicular growth, which is monitored via blood work and pelvic ultrasonography usually every 2 to 3 days. Once the ovarian follicles are deemed ready, an oocyte maturation trigger is administered (GnRHa and/or compounded human chorionic gonadotropins) after which a transvaginal or transabdominal oocyte needle aspiration is performed within 34 to 36 hours under monitored sedation. Retrieved oocytes are transported to the embryology laboratory to be assessed under the microscope to determine maturity. Mature oocytes undergo either cryopreservation or in vitro fertilization for embryo creation if a sperm source is available from a sexually intimate partner or donor (anonymous or known). Immature oocytes are discarded or cryopreserved in hopes of future in vitro maturation when the technology is developed. Fertilized oocytes are cultured over the course of 7 days and embryos are cryopreserved upon reaching a blastocyst stage. Both mature oocytes and embryos may be cryopreserved indefinitely. When the patient is ready to procreate, the mature oocytes or embryos are thawed. Thawed mature oocytes undergo in vitro fertilization for embryo creation as they would have when fresh prior to cryopreservation. Last, embryos are transferred to a uterine-retaining individual (self, partner, or gestation carrier) in order to attempt pregnancy.[47] Although family building from mature oocyte cryopreservation has been demonstrated in transmasculine individuals, patients should understand that counseling is limited by the lack of data on the long-term impact of testosterone on reproductive capacity and reported oocyte thaw outcomes in this population.[48,49]

If masculinizing hormones are started prior to FP, mature oocyte or embryo cryopreservation remains an option. Transmasculine individuals have traditionally been asked to temporarily stop testosterone prior to controlled ovarian stimulation for a predetermined period of time, though the ideal length of discontinuation remains unknown.[50] However, studies in animal models suggest that testosterone only compromises quantity and not quality of oocytes. Oocyte quantity may improve with even a short washout period but could be permanently low in long-term testosterone use. These studies suggest that controlled ovarian stimulation is possible even while on testosterone as oocyte quality is unaffected, but a washout period will optimize oocyte quantity.[51,52] Best practice should include shared decision-making to determine if and when testosterone should be paused given the potential psychological and/or physical stress on TGD individuals. A washout period of at least 3 month is usually recommended, but shorter periods such as 1 month are acceptable if stopping testosterone poses difficulty. Individuals may resume testosterone immediately after oocyte aspiration or await onset of menses to avoid an irregular menstrual pattern.

For transmasculine individuals desiring GAS, the potential loss of reproductive organs should be considered. In the case of oophorectomy, partial or complete loss of ovarian tissue may limit or render impossible to obtain mature oocytes for future genetically related children. In the case of hysterectomy, there will be a need for a gestation carrier when ready to procreate.

OPTIONS FOR FERTILITY PRESERVATION IN TRANSGENDER AND GENDER DIVERSE PEOPLE ASSIGNED MALE AT BIRTH

For prepubertal transfeminine individuals starting pubertal blockers (such as GnRHa) followed by feminizing hormones (antiandrogens such as spironolactone or CPA combined with estrogen), the longer term hormonal effects on testicular tissue and sperm development may lead to loss of reproductive function.[50] Unlike ovarian tissue cryopreservation, testicular tissue or spermatogonial stem cell cryopreservation remains experimental with successful outcomes only reported in animal models.[53] Testicular tissue cryopreservation programs have emerged around the world primarily in the context of prepubertal cismale patients with cancer [54] with limited thaw and transplantation data. Therefore, the most ideal FP option for transfeminine individuals is sperm cryopreservation prior to feminizing therapy; however, this would require individuals to await puberty. The process of sperm cryopreservation (or sperm freezing) involves obtaining a sperm sample usually via masturbation. If erection or ejaculation is not possible for sperm collection, there are assistive ejaculatory methods such as electroejaculation and penile vibratory stimulation. Other nonejaculatory sperm collection techniques include surgical testicular or epididymal sperm aspiration. If GAHT is initiated prior to FP, sperm cryopreservation remains an option for individuals who are willing to temporarily discontinue feminizing hormones. Discontinuation will result in endogenous testosterone production which can pose psychological and/or physical stress on TGD individuals. The ideal length of time for antiandrogen and estrogen discontinuation remains unknown,[54] and deciding how to proceed requires shared decision-making as for transmasculine individuals on masculinizing hormones. Sperm can be cryopreserved indefinitely. When the patient is ready to procreate, the sperm is thawed and used for artificial insemination of a uterine-retaining individual or in vitro fertilization with matured oocytes from a partner or donor (anonymous or known). Artificial insemination or in vitro fertilization is possible if specific sperm parameters are met including a required total motility count threshold. Last, embryos are transferred to any uterine-retaining individual (partner or gestation carrier) in order to attempt pregnancy.

CONTRACEPTION

While GAHT may suppress gonadal function, it is not a reliable method for contraception. Pregnancy prevention counseling is necessary for all sexually active TGD individuals who do not wish to reproduce and retain the ability to become pregnant or impregnate others.[55] The provider must have an open discussion with the individual on sexual orientation and preferences in order to identify an appropriate contraceptive method. Special considerations include different side effect profiles, barriers to accessing care, and misconceptions regarding reproduction in the TGD population. However, many providers often lack the appropriate training and feel unprepared to provide this care. The Society of Family Planning along with leading experts in the field of contraception have recognized the need to standardize contraceptive care for TGD individuals and published detailed clinical opinions and guidelines that are readily available.[56,57] For transmasculine individuals, a decrease in fertility may occur but conception is still possible even if amenorrheic from active testosterone use. Testosterone is also known to have irreversible teratogenic effects on the developing fetus.[19] Therefore, concurrent use of hormonal contraception and testosterone is recommended for transmasculine individuals. Any chosen contraceptive method is acceptable as there are no contraindications with testosterone. Most transmasculine individuals will opt for progestin-only methods (such as the levonorgestrel intrauterine device, etonogestrel implant, or depot medroxyprogesterone acetate injection) to avoid any estrogenic changes.[55] For transfeminine individuals, complete azoospermia is not always achieved from active estrogen use; therefore, barrier contraception or other reliable contraceptive method should be used if sexually active with a cisgender individual.[19]

Last, all TGD individuals should be counseled on safe sex practices as a means of sexually transmitted infection prevention.

SUMMARY

While an essential component of gender-affirming care, hormone therapies impact reproductive potential. Studies show that nearly 50% of TGD individuals express a desire for future children[3] and more than 70% think about FP, though only a minority pursues it.[7] Common barriers to pursing FP include cost, lack of proper counseling, and an individual's desire to proceed with gender-affirming treatment without any further delay. To mitigate these barriers, the ASRM joins the WAPATH and the Endocrine Society in strongly recommending that all TGD individuals be counseled regarding fertility prior to initiating medical and/or surgical gender-affirming treatments.[12] The goal of the fertility consultation should be to discuss reproductive potential after transitioning and strategize for future family building if desired. Existing options for future reproduction include gonadal tissue cryopreservation (for prepubertal individuals), gametes or embryo cryopreservation (for postpubertal individuals), third party reproduction (such as donor sperm/mature oocytes and gestational carrier), and adoption. A multidisciplinary approach to care throughout the process of FP is necessary as individuals, particularly adolescents and young adults are at increased risk for psychological and physical distress due to gender incongruent experiences. FP should be individualized based on the timing, type, and duration of gender-affirming treatments. While there have been advances in the technology and standardization of reproductive health care for TGD individuals, many gaps remain in our knowledge which require further research and evidence-based approaches to caring for this population.

CLINIC CARE POINTS

- Counseling regarding fertility should be done at each stage of transition, including before medical and surgical transition and before pubertal suppression in adolescents.
- While GAHT may suppress gonadal function, it is not a reliable method for contraception.

DISCLOSURES

The authors have nothing to disclose.

REFERENCES

1. How many adults and youth identify as transgender in the United States? Los Angeles: Williams Institute; 2022.
2. Winter S, Diamond M, Green J, et al. Transgender people: health at the margins of society. Lancet 2016;388(10042):390–400.
3. Wierckx K, Van Caenegem E, Pennings G, et al. Reproductive wish in transsexual men. Hum Reprod 2012;27(2):483–7.
4. Chen D, Matson M, Macapagal K, et al. Attitudes toward fertility and reproductive health among transgender and gender-nonconforming adolescents. J Adolesc Health 2018;63(1):62–8.
5. Hembree WC, Cohen-Kettenis PT, Gooren L, et al. Endocrine treatment of gender-dysphoric/gender-incongruent persons: an endocrine society clinical practice guideline. J Clin Endocrinol Metab 2017;102(11):3869–903.

6. Alpern S, Yaish I, Wagner-Kolasko G, et al. Why fertility preservation rates of transgender men are much lower than those of transgender women. Reprod Biomed Online 2022;44(5):943–50.

7. Auer MK, Fuss J, Nieder TO, et al. Desire to have children among transgender people in germany: a cross-sectional multi-center study. J Sex Med 2018;15(5):757–67.

8. Nahata L, Tishelman AC, Caltabellotta NM, et al. Low fertility preservation utilization among transgender youth. J Adolesc Health 2017;61(1):40–4.

9. Chen D, Simons L, Johnson EK, et al. Fertility preservation for transgender adolescents. J Adolesc Health 2017;61(1):120–3.

10. Defreyne J, Van Schuylenbergh J, Motmans J, et al. Parental desire and fertility preservation in assigned female at birth transgender people living in Belgium. Fertil Steril 2020;113(1):149–57.e142.

11. Vyas N, Douglas CR, Mann C, et al. Access, barriers, and decisional regret in pursuit of fertility preservation among transgender and gender-diverse individuals. Fertil Steril 2021;115(4):1029–34.

12. Access to fertility services by transgender and nonbinary persons: an Ethics Committee opinion. Fertil Steril 2021;115(4):874–8.

13. Coleman E, Radix AE, Bouman WP, et al. Standards of care for the health of transgender and gender diverse people, version 8. Int J Transgend Health 2022;23(Suppl 1):S1–259.

14. Jindarak S, Nilprapha K, Atikankul T, et al. Spermatogenesis abnormalities following hormonal therapy in transwomen. BioMed Res Int 2018;2018:7919481.

15. Kent MA, Winoker JS, Grotas AB. Effects of feminizing hormones on sperm production and malignant changes: microscopic examination of post orchiectomy specimens in transwomen. Urology 2018;121:93–6.

16. Jiang DD, Swenson E, Mason M, et al. Effects of estrogen on spermatogenesis in transgender women. Urology 2019;132:117–22.

17. Matoso A, Khandakar B, Yuan S, et al. Spectrum of findings in orchiectomy specimens of persons undergoing gender confirmation surgery. Hum Pathol 2018;76:91–9.

18. Vereecke G, Defreyne J, Van Saen D, et al. Characterisation of testicular function and spermatogenesis in transgender women. Hum Reprod 2021;36(1):5–15.

19. Sinha A, Mei L, Ferrando C. The effect of estrogen therapy on spermatogenesis in transgender women. F S Rep 2021;2(3):347–51.

20. Lübbert H, Leo-Rossberg I, Hammerstein J. Effects of ethinyl estradiol on semen quality and various hormonal parameters in a eugonadal male. Fertil Steril 1992;58(3):603–8.

21. Mattawanon N, Spencer JB, Schirmer DA 3rd, et al. Fertility preservation options in transgender people: A review. Rev Endocr Metab Disord 2018;19(3):231–42.

22. de Nie I, van Mello NM, Vlahakis E, et al. Successful restoration of spermatogenesis following gender-affirming hormone therapy in transgender women. Cell Rep Med 2023;4(1):100858.

23. Alford AV, Theisen KM, Kim N, et al. Successful ejaculatory sperm cryopreservation after cessation of long-term estrogen therapy in a transgender female. Urology 2020;136:e48–50.

24. Adeleye AJ, Reid G, Kao CN, et al. Semen parameters among transgender women with a history of hormonal treatment. Urology 2019;124:136–41.

25. T'Sjoen G, Arcelus J, Gooren L, et al. Endocrinology of transgender medicine. Endocr Rev 2019;40(1):97–117.

26. Loverro G, Resta L, Dellino M, et al. Uterine and ovarian changes during testosterone administration in young female-to-male transsexuals. Taiwan J Obstet Gynecol 2016;55(5):686–91.

27. Light AD, Obedin-Maliver J, Sevelius JM, et al. Transgender men who experienced pregnancy after female-to-male gender transitioning. Obstet Gynecol 2014;124(6):1120–7.

28. Caanen MR, Schouten NE, Kuijper EAM, et al. Effects of long-term exogenous testosterone administration on ovarian morphology, determined by transvaginal (3D) ultrasound in female-to-male transsexuals. Hum Reprod 2017;32(7):1457–64.

29. Ikeda K, Baba T, Noguchi H, et al. Excessive androgen exposure in female-to-male transsexual persons of reproductive age induces hyperplasia of the ovarian cortex and stroma but not polycystic ovary morphology. Hum Reprod 2013;28(2): 453–61.

30. Borrás A, Manau MD, Fabregues F, et al. Endocrinological and ovarian histological investigations in assigned female at birth transgender people undergoing testosterone therapy. Reprod Biomed Online 2021;43(2):289–97.

31. Grimstad FW, Fowler KG, New EP, et al. Uterine pathology in transmasculine persons on testosterone: a retrospective multicenter case series. Am J Obstet Gynecol 2019;220(3):257.e251–7.

32. Hawkins M, Deutsch MB, Obedin-Maliver J, et al. Endometrial findings among transgender and gender nonbinary people using testosterone at the time of gender-affirming hysterectomy. Fertil Steril 2021;115(5):1312–7.

33. Leung A, Sakkas D, Pang S, et al. Assisted reproductive technology outcomes in female-to-male transgender patients compared with cisgender patients: a new frontier in reproductive medicine. Fertil Steril 2019;112(5):858–65.

34. Adeleye AJ, Cedars MI, Smith J, et al. Ovarian stimulation for fertility preservation or family building in a cohort of transgender men. J Assist Reprod Genet 2019; 36(10):2155–61.

35. Amir H, Yaish I, Samara N, et al. Ovarian stimulation outcomes among transgender men compared with fertile cisgender women. J Assist Reprod Genet 2020;37(10):2463–72.

36. Ghofranian A, Estevez SL, Gellman C, et al. Fertility treatment outcomes in transgender men with a history of testosterone therapy. F S Rep 2023;4(4):367–74.

37. Barrero JA, Mockus I. Preservation of fertility in transgender men on long-term testosterone therapy: a systematic review of oocyte retrieval outcomes during and after exogenous androgen exposure. Transgend Health 2023;8(5):408–19.

38. Lee JY. Puberty assessment and consideration of gonadotropin-releasing hormone agonists in transgender and gender-diverse youth. Pediatr Ann 2023;52(12): e462–6.

39. Salas-Humara C, Sequeira GM, Rossi W, et al. Gender affirming medical care of transgender youth. Curr Probl Pediatr Adolesc Health Care 2019;49(9):100683.

40. Bertelloni S, Baroncelli GI, Ferdeghini M, et al. Final height, gonadal function and bone mineral density of adolescent males with central precocious puberty after therapy with gonadotropin-releasing hormone analogues. Eur J Pediatr 2000; 159(5):369–74.

41. Pasquino AM, Pucarelli I, Accardo F, et al. Long-term observation of 87 girls with idiopathic central precocious puberty treated with gonadotropin-releasing hormone analogs: impact on adult height, body mass index, bone mineral content, and reproductive function. J Clin Endocrinol Metab 2008;93(1):190–5.

42. Zaliznyak M, Yuan N, Bresee C, et al. How early in life do transgender adults begin to experience gender dysphoria? why this matters for patients, providers, and for our healthcare system. Sex Med 2021;9(6):100448.
43. Fertility preservation in patients undergoing gonadotoxic therapy or gonadectomy: a committee opinion. Fertil Steril 2019;112(6):1022–33.
44. Insogna IG, Ginsburg E, Srouji S. Fertility preservation for adolescent transgender male patients: a case series. J Adolesc Health 2020;66(6):750–3.
45. Rothenberg SS, Witchel SF, Menke MN. Oocyte cryopreservation in a transgender male adolescent. N Engl J Med 2019;380(9):886–7.
46. Smitz J, Dolmans MM, Donnez J, et al. Current achievements and future research directions in ovarian tissue culture, in vitro follicle development and transplantation: implications for fertility preservation. Hum Reprod Update 2010;16(4):395–414.
47. Blakemore JK, Quinn GP, Fino ME. A discussion of options, outcomes, and future recommendations for fertility preservation for transmasculine individuals. Urol Clin North Am 2019;46(4):495–503.
48. Barrett F, Shaw J, Blakemore JK, et al. Fertility preservation for adolescent and young adult transmen: a case series and insights on oocyte cryopreservation. Front Endocrinol 2022;13:873508.
49. Maxwell S, Noyes N, Keefe D, et al. Pregnancy outcomes after fertility preservation in transgender men. Obstet Gynecol 2017;129(6):1031–4.
50. Neblett MF 2nd, Hipp HS. Fertility considerations in transgender persons. Endocrinol Metab Clin North Am 2019;48(2):391–402.
51. Schwartz AR, Xu M, Henderson NC, et al. Impaired in vitro fertilization outcomes following testosterone treatment improve with washout in a mouse model of gender-affirming hormone treatment. Am J Obstet Gynecol 2023;229(4):419 e411–e419 e410.
52. Dela Cruz C, Wandoff A, Brunette M, et al. In vitro fertilization outcomes in a mouse model of gender-affirming hormone therapy in transmasculine youth. F S Sci 2023;4(4):302–10.
53. Kabiri D, Safrai M, Gropp M, et al. Establishment of a controlled slow freezing-based approach for experimental clinical cryopreservation of human prepubertal testicular tissues. F S Rep 2022;3(1):47–56.
54. Moussaoui D, Surbone A, Adam C, et al. Testicular tissue cryopreservation for fertility preservation in prepubertal and adolescent boys: A 6 year experience from a Swiss multi-center network. Front Pediatr 2022;10:909000.
55. ACOG Committee Opinion No. 823, Health care for transgender and gender diverse individuals: correction. Obstet Gynecol 2022;139(2):345.
56. Bonnington A, Dianat S, Kerns J, et al. Society of Family Planning clinical recommendations: Contraceptive counseling for transgender and gender diverse people who were female sex assigned at birth. Contraception 2020;102(2):70–82.
57. Krempasky C, Harris M, Abern L, et al. Contraception across the transmasculine spectrum. Am J Obstet Gynecol 2020;222(2):134–43.

Lipid Disorders and Pregnancy

Daria Schatoff, MD[a], Irene Y. Jung, BA[a], Ira J. Goldberg, MD[b,c],*

KEYWORDS

- Cholesterol • Triglyceride • Estrogen • LDL • Chylomicron • Pancreatitis
- Pregnancy • Hyperlipidemia

KEY POINTS

- Hypertriglyceridemia is exacerbated with pregnancy.
- Hypertriglyceridemic pancreatitis is most frequent in the third trimester.
- Although the use of statins during pregnancy should be avoided, toxic effects of these drugs have not been confirmed.
- Marked hypercholesterolemia could lead to cardiovascular issues during pregnancy.

INTRODUCTION

Lipid disorders occasionally complicate infertility treatments and the course of a pregnancy and affect the use of medications during lactation. The most dramatic situation is the development of pancreatitis during pregnancy, which sometimes occurs in patients without previously known hyperlipidemia. Another issue to consider is cardiovascular risk and the maintenance of therapies in patients with known genetic hypercholesterolemia previously treated prior to pregnancy. Finally, this review addresses the risks for the developing fetus and newborn due to the presence and treatment of lipid disorders in the mother.

All lipoproteins contain a core of hydrophobic, that is not water soluble, lipids surrounded by a coat of phospholipids and proteins that are amphipathic, being able to interact with both hydrophobic and hydrophilic molecules, thus allowing triglycerides and cholesteryl esters to remain in the solution. Triglycerides circulate as a component of 2 large lipoproteins: chylomicrons and very low-density lipoproteins (VLDLs). Chylomicrons, the larger of these particles, contain dietary triglycerides that are assembled in enterocytes, secreted into the lymph, and enter the circulation

[a] New York University Grossman School of Medicine, New York, USA; [b] Department of Medicine, New York University Grossman School of Medicine, New York, USA; [c] Holman Division of Endocrinology, Diabetes & Metabolism, New York University Grossman School of Medicine, New York, USA
* Corresponding author.
E-mail address: Ira.Goldberg@nyulangone.org

Endocrinol Metab Clin N Am 53 (2024) 483–495
https://doi.org/10.1016/j.ecl.2024.05.009
0889-8529/24/© 2024 Elsevier Inc. All rights reserved, including those for text and data mining, AI training, and similar technologies.

when the lymphatic duct empties into the right subclavian artery. VLDLs are secreted from the liver and carry triglycerides assembled from newly synthesized fatty acids made from carbohydrates and some amino acids, and fatty acids obtained from lipoprotein and nonesterified fatty acids captured by the liver. Both chylomicrons and VLDL interact with lipoprotein lipase attached to the luminal surface of capillary endothelial cells. The larger chylomicrons are more likely to hit the wall of the capillaries and interact with the lipase leading to a much shorter plasma half-life. Chylomicrons lose greater than 50% of their triglycerides, which are converted to nonesterified fatty acids and monoglycerides, during lipolysis. The released lipid becomes the substrate for adenine triphosphate (ATP) production by the heart and skeletal muscles and for storage in adipose. The remaining lipid and protein, in what is now called a remnant, is primarily cleared by the liver. VLDL triglycerides undergo a similar fate, but the remaining particle is eventually converted to the cholesterol-rich and atherogenic low-density lipoproteins (LDLs). The competition of these 2 particles for lipoprotein lipase is the reason that elevations of VLDL above 500 mg/dL, the saturation level of the enzyme, can lead to fasting hyperchylomicronemia. Several additional factors regulate triglyceride metabolism and will be discussed later and are reviewed in more detail elsewhere.[1]

The 2 cholesterol-rich particles, LDLs and high-density lipoproteins (HDLs), are smaller and therefore denser than the triglyceride particles. Approximately two-thirds of the cholesterol is esterified to the hydroxyl group in the 3 position of the A ring, reducing its charge and allowing it to position within the lipoprotein core. Likely in humans, both LDL and HDL are capable of delivering cholesterol to steroidogenic tissues. Lipoprotein deficiencies do not lead to defects in adrenal or gonadal hormones as these tissues also can synthesize cholesterol if needed. Patients with abetalipoproteinemia do not have pregnancy issues provided they receive large supplemental doses of fat-soluble vitamins.[2] LDL levels are regulated by synthesis, conversion from VLDL, and uptake by the liver LDL receptor (LDLR). Other factors regulating LDL and the LDLR are discussed in the section on familial hypercholesterolemia (FH). HDLs are synthesized by the liver and intestines. HDLs obtain additional lipid that is transferred during lipolysis of triglyceride-rich lipoproteins and also from release of cholesterol from cells such as macrophages.

HYPERTRIGLYCERIDEMIA IN PREGNANCY

The most concerning lipid disorder that can complicate pregnancy is the development of severe hypertriglyceridemia leading to pancreatitis. This is especially a concern in women with genetic disorders affecting lipoprotein lipase actions: a condition referred to as familial chylomicron syndrome (FCS). Often FCS has been diagnosed during childhood but sometimes it is first identified in young women when they are given birth control pills or have lipids checked during pregnancy. Genetic testing for defects in lipoprotein lipase, its endothelial cell binding protein (GPIHBP1), an intracellular adaptor (LMF1), apolipoprotein (Apo) A5 (which prevents inactivation of the lipase), and the lipase coactivator ApoC2 are readily available. As new therapies are being developed (see later discussion), it is likely these genetic tests will be performed on all patients with triglyceride levels greater than 500 mg/dL. Homozygous defects in lipoprotein lipase pathway genes are relatively rare, totaling approximately 1/500,000, but they are more common in specific populations such as French Canadians.[3] For this reason, the chances of a baby inheriting FCS are very low. Patients with heterozygous mutations can also present with pregnancy-associated hypertriglyceridemia and pancreatitis, especially if the second contributing cause of hypertriglyceridemia is present such as diabetes or obesity. Another consideration is the impact of hypertriglyceridemia on pre-eclamptic pregnancies and preterm deliveries. A cross-sectional study by Belo noted higher mean serum triglyceride concentration in pre-eclamptic women when compared to healthy pregnant women.[4] Women with spontaneous preterm births were noted to have elevated triglycerides and cholesterol levels prior to 15 weeks' gestation, when compared to women with term births.[5]

Pregnancy Increases Triglyceride Levels

Estrogens stimulate hepatic triglyceride production and therefore increase circulating VLDL levels.[6] Although the exact mechanism for this is not totally understood, rodent studies indicate the estrogens will block insulin-mediated ApoB degradation.[7] Estrogen also markedly reduces a second lipase enzyme, hepatic lipase.[8] Hepatic lipase will degrade triglycerides in smaller VLDL and is, in part, the reason for the increase in HDL with estrogen as it decreases HDL catabolism.

Pancreatitis Leads to an Increase in Fetal Loss

In one recent meta-analysis from the United Kingdom, pancreatitis was associated with approximately 3% maternal mortality and 12.3% fetal loss.[9] This maternal death rate is similar to that of pancreatitis in nonpregnant patients. Fetal loss was highest with pancreatitis during the first trimester, presumably most were due to gallbladder disease. The majority of pancreatitis cases, almost two-third, were in the third trimester, a time when hypertriglyceridemia becomes most severe; however, the highest rate of fetal death was in the first trimester. Therefore, while the exact numbers are not available, it appears that fetal loss is likely increased with hypertriglyceridemic pancreatitis. Another meta-analysis noted that reports from eastern Asia had a higher percent of hypertriglyceridemia as a cause of pancreatitis during pregnancy.[10]

The high risk of pancreatitis in women with FCS has led some to use surrogate carriers. Other women with FCS have chosen to carry their own pregnancies. Pregnant women with FCS should have their triglyceride levels carefully monitored; obtaining weekly triglyceride levels, especially during the third trimester, is appropriate. If triglyceride levels exceed 2000 mg/dL, the level thought to be necessary to induce pancreatitis,[11] pregnancies are often terminated; this is a risk/benefit decision that includes the mother's response to an extraordinarily restricted diet of almost no fat or free carbohydrates (sweets, bread, rice, pasta, and potatoes). There are cases where weekly or twice a week plasmapheresis has been used to extend the pregnancy.[12,13] For non-FCS patients, better control of diabetes, if present, and dietary modifications should reduce triglyceride levels.

Preventive Strategies

Preventive strategies are often the best approach to prevent triglyceride-induced pancreatitis. Although not recommended as a routine screening procedure, patients with a background risk of developing severe hypertriglyceridemia should have a lipid panel—triglyceride, cholesterol, HDL, and calculated LDL—before or early in the pregnancy. These include patients with obesity, type 2 diabetes, or polycystic ovarian syndrome (PCOS). In patients with increased risk, case reports have described pancreatitis due to the estrogen surge during an in vitro fertilization cycle.[14,15] Such patients should be diet-restricted and encouraged to exercise.

Lactation

Lactation is not an issue in patients with hypertriglyceridemia, even due to FCS. After birth, triglyceride levels usually decrease, and pancreatitis is less of an issue. Although it has been reported that milk from patients with FCS has reduced amounts of fat and is therefore lower calorie, it is unclear whether the lower fat content of breast milk is due to the enzyme defect leading to less mammary fat production or the low-calorie diet eaten by these patients. Studies in genetically modified mice have shown no defect in either fat or vitamin A content of milk from lipoprotein lipase knockout mice.[16]

Pharmacologic Treatments

Pharmacologic treatments are useful in severe hypertriglyceridemia during pregnancy. Both high-dose omega-3 fatty acids and fibric acid drugs, such as gemfibrozil and fenofibrate, have been given to pregnant women without obvious side effects.[17] It is unlikely that these medications are effective in patients with FCS.[18] As discussed later, statins, which are less effective for triglyceride reduction, should be avoided. New approaches to triglyceride reduction include molecular methods to block liver production of ApoC3, an inhibitor of lipoprotein lipase and liver uptake of triglyceride-rich lipoproteins, and angiopoietin-like protein 3 (ANGPTL3), another lipase inhibitor.[19]

HYPERCHOLESTEROLEMIA AND PREGNANCY

Another concerning lipid disorder that complicates pregnancy is FH or elevated levels of LDL. Increased LDL levels could result from either excessive liver lipoprotein production or defective plasma clearance of LDL. Overproduction can present as combined hyperlipidemia, increased cholesterol and triglyceride due to greater circulating levels of VLDL and LDL. LDL clearance from the bloodstream primarily is mediated by the LDLR. Apo B, the major structural protein of VLDL and LDL, binds to the LDLR leading to hepatic LDL uptake, delivery of LDL to the lysosome, and recycling of the receptor to the cell surface. Statins and proprotein convertase subtilisin/kexin type 9 (PCSK9) inhibitors reduce LDL levels by increasing hepatic LDLR levels.

Genetics of Hypercholesterolemia

FH is most often due to loss-of-function mutations in the LDLR gene; LDLR mutations account for around 86% to 88% of FH cases.[20] Less common causes of FH include defects in the LDL binding region of ApoB,[20] mutations of intracellular proteins required for normal LDL recycling, and gain-of-function mutations in PCSK9 leading to more LDLR degradation.[21,22] Loss-of-function PCSK9 variants actually offer a protective effect in individuals predisposed to higher LDL cholesterol (LDL-C) levels.[23–25] ApoE also serves as a ligand for the LDLR and other lipoprotein receptors. It has 3 genetic variants; in some patients, ApoE2/E2 leads to dysbetalipoproteinemia, a condition that may present with increases in both cholesterol and triglyceride due to the accumulation of cholesterol-rich VLDL or with only increased triglyceride or LDL, thus mimicking FH.[26–28]

FH is an autosomal dominant genetic disorder that leads to greater risk for development of premature atherosclerotic cardiovascular disease (ASCVD).[29] Heterozygous FH (HeFH), due to one copy of the affected gene, is fairly common affecting around 1 in 311 people; thus, it is one of the most common genetic abnormalities found in the general population. FH is underdiagnosed and undertreated with less than 1% being diagnosed.[30–32] This underdiagnosis may be especially common in young women who often have not had a lipid profile. Homozygous FH (HoFH), due to 2 copies of the affected gene, is quite rare. The Orphanet rare disease database estimates HoFH to occur in about 3 in every 1,000,000 individuals.[33] Other recent studies, however, have reported that HoFH may actually occur in about 1 in 170,000 to 300,000 individuals.[34,35] HeFH is clinically diagnosed when LDL-C reaches levels of ≥160 mg/dL in children and ≥190 in adults with evidence of gene defects or affected relatives. Clinical criteria for HoFH are LDL-C levels of ≥400 mg/dL with one or both parents diagnosed with HeFH,[36] extensor tendon xanthomas, corneal arcus, and early-onset ASCVD.[36] Because HoFH and severe HeFH associate with both ischemic heart disease and aortic valve disease, these patients may need to consult a cardiologist.

While the nature of this relationship is not yet clear, correlative studies have shown that increases in 17β-estradiol and progesterone as well as insulin are associated with increases in ApoB and LDL-C levels.[37,38] Additional studies have also demonstrated that there is an associated increase in hepatic lipase activity and decrease in lipoprotein lipase activity during pregnancy, which could explain increased circulating lipid levels.[39]

Fertility and Fetal Health

A clear link between FH and infertility has yet to be fully delineated. A 2011 study by Toleikyte and colleagues with 1093 FH women showed that fertility rates between women with FH and without FH were similar.[40] However, several recent studies showed an association between dyslipidemia and infertility, which could potentially affect FH women. Preconception high LDL and low HDL levels have been associated with decreased fecundability by 19% to 32%.[41,42] Complicating this analysis is also the dyslipidemia associated with PCOS.

The same study by Toleikyte and colleagues found that frequency of preterm birth, low birth weight, and congenital malformations were all similar in women with FH when compared to women without FH.[40] This study also showed no associated increased risk of preterm birth, low birth weight, and congenital malformations with increasing LDL levels.[40] Therefore, pregnancy in women with FH appears to be safe for both mothers and babies.

Lipoprotein(a) and Thrombosis

Lipoprotein(a) [Lp(a)] is a type of LDL that is a significant risk factor for cardiovascular disease events, such as myocardial infarction, stroke, and aortic stenosis.[43,44] It has also been found to be more prevalent in individuals with FH than in the general population, affecting around an estimated 30% to 50% of individuals with HeFH.[45,46] Additionally, in individuals with FH and elevated Lp(a) levels, there is approximately 2 fold increase in risk of ASCVD compared to individuals with only FH.[47]

In recent years, a topic of contention is whether Lp(a) promotes thrombosis. Owing to its structural homology with plasminogen, it has been thought to compete with plasminogen for its endothelial cell receptor, which is required to form cleavage-activated plasmin, an important player in the degradation of fibrin clots. This competition was thought to contribute to venous thrombosis, and potential associations were described in several studies.[48] However, in several clinical observational studies, Lp(a) was not a predictive risk factor for venous thrombosis, unless at very high Lp(a) values of greater than 95th percentile.[49,50]

To prevent thrombosis, aspirin is often used as a simpler and more inexpensive alternative to anticoagulants for both primary and secondary thrombosis prophylaxis in nonpregnant patients. Several studies have shown that consistent use of low-dose aspirin of 100 mg daily effectively reduces recurrent episodes of venous thromboembolism (VTE).[51,52] Additionally, a study by Matharu and colleagues showed that effectiveness of aspirin is comparable to that of other anticoagulants and there was no statistically significant difference in risk of VTE or adverse events.[53] Whether aspirin prophylaxis should be prescribed for pregnant patients with very high levels of Lp(a) without a clinical history of thromboembolic disease is unclear. Of note, one study associated high Lp(a) levels with greater than 2 fold greater incidence of pre-eclampsia and stillborn babies.[54] Lp(a) levels can be reduced by apheresis as well as using not yet approved antisense[55] and silencing RNA[56] therapies. These options could be considered in women with very high risk for complications and history of recurrent pregnancy loss.

LIPID-LOWERING DRUG THERAPY DURING PREGNANCY

Two therapeutic dilemmas are when to begin treatment of hypercholesterolemia in women of childbearing age and whether to continue those treatments during pregnancy. For HoFH, there is no question that treatment is indicated as these patients can develop ASCVD during childhood. For them, the issue is the choice of an agent, as usually LDL reducing medications require upregulation of the LDLR. HeFH can also lead to ASCVD in women of childbearing age. They are usually treated with statins, as earlier treatment is better. In 2019, a 20 year follow-up study of 214 children with FH via LDLR or ApoB mutation and a modest 32% decrease in LDL showed that earlier treatment with statins significantly reduced cardiovascular events.[57] Young women with high levels of Lp(a) and other risk factors, especially family history, are also likely to be treated with statins. PCSK9 inhibitors, which lower LDL 50% to 60%, are also used in HeFH and should reduce ASCVD risk further.[58] These therapies for LDL reduction are rapidly advancing, with silencing RNA to PCSK9 and, in clinical trials, the use of CRISPR technology. For HoFH, monoclonal antibodies to ANGPTL3 are currently the US Food and Drug Administration (FDA)-approved because they have led to a marked reduction in circulating LDL levels.[59] There are reports of the use of plasma apheresis to lower LDL in pregnant women with FH and, as noted earlier, to reduce hypertriglyceridemia in women with FCS.[60]

Statin Safety During Pregnancy

Historically, statins have been designated category X by the FDA, indicating risk of fetal abnormalities in animal or human investigation. This label was imparted during initial toxicity studies of statins in rats and rabbits, which revealed skeletal abnormalities with exposure to lovastatin. Of note, these abnormalities could be reversed by coadministration of mevalonate, the product of hydroxy-3-methyl-glutaryl-coenzyme A A (HMG-CoA) reductase.[61] For these reasons, statins are contraindicated in pregnancy and lactation. Although the evidence for statin use in pregnancy does not reveal major hazards, it also does not indicate safety. Thus, the use of statins is cautioned against given concern that potential risks to the fetus do not outweigh benefits. Statins are metabolized rapidly; thus, it is reasonable to stop them when pregnancy is attempted.

A number of studies have examined safety and pregnancy outcomes in women exposed to statins. These studies were further prompted by the trend of childbearing occurring later in life, when more women may have higher risk for cardiovascular disease and thus more exposure to statin therapy. A systematic review by Kusters and colleagues examined teratogenic effects of statin exposure in pregnancy in both humans and animals. No consistent pattern of congenital abnormalities was observed in humans, and conflicting results were noted in animal studies. When congenital abnormalities occurred, these were observed in rodents receiving excessive doses of statins.[62] Similarly, a meta-analysis by Zarek did not signal harm with statin use in pregnancy. However, it was noted that women exposed to statins had higher risk of miscarriage and were more likely to undergo elective termination.[63] It was postulated that the increased risk of miscarriage reflected maternal morbidity rather than an effect of statin therapy itself, as statin use implies older age or higher metabolic risk.

A systemic review by Karalis and colleagues of human studies again did not demonstrate a clear relationship between statin use and pregnancy. Although the evidence was conflicting and not conclusive enough to assure safety, there was no quality evidence to support terminating a pregnancy because of potential risk of congenital abnormalities from statin exposure.[64] Overall, women who are exposed to statins while pregnant should undergo screening for congenital abnormalities in utero; this is a precaution as risk for abnormalities is unlikely to be increased.[65] Currently, studies on statins and breastfeeding are quite limited. However, some studies show that there is relatively little transfer of statins into breast milk, and the benefits of continuing statins during breastfeeding may outweigh the risks.[66]

Fibrates and Pancreatitis Risk

Fibrates agonize transcription factor peroxisome proliferator-activated receptor-alpha, increase lipoprotein lipase-mediated catabolism of VLDL, and decrease ApoB and VLDL production. They are designated as category C during pregnancy. Although animal studies did not demonstrate congenital abnormalities, these studies were too small to confide safety.[67] In humans, case reports of select women with severe hypertriglyceridemia at risk of pancreatitis receiving gemfibrozil therapy did not show clear adverse effects or fetal abnormalities.[68] The National Lipid Association recommends that women with elevated triglycerides greater than 500 mg/dL can be managed with lifestyle modifications and omega-3 fatty acids or with fenofibrate or gemfibrozil early in the second trimester based on clinical judgment and that these agents may be used during lactation (grade B recommendation).[69] It is unknown whether fibrates are present in breast milk.

Fish Oil

Omega-3 fatty acids reduce hepatic triglyceride synthesis and increase fatty acid oxidation in the liver and skeletal muscle. They are designated category C. Adverse outcomes from exposure appear unlikely. A randomized double-blind randomized placebo-controlled trial of 98 pregnant women receiving fish oil supplementation from 20 weeks gestation to delivery did not demonstrate adverse effects.[70] Omega-3 fatty acids are present in breast milk.

Resins

Cholestyramine and colesevelam bind bile acids in the intestine. This creates an insoluble complex with both biliary and dietary cholesterol leading to greater cholesterol excretion in the feces and decreased serum LDL levels. It is designated category B, indicating no risk in animal studies. In rat and rabbit studies receiving colesevelam hydrochloride, no evidence of maternal or fetal toxicity was found.[71] Given its lack of systemic absorption, it is unlikely to be present in breast milk. Since resins interfere with vitamin absorption, providing additional vitamin supplementation is reasonable. The National Lipid Association recommends that women taking lipid-lowering medications prior to pregnancy, all, except bile acid sequestrants, should be stopped when the women become pregnant, or are trying to become pregnant (grade B recommendation).[69]

Bempedoic acid, an inhibitor of citrate lyase, an enzyme involved in cholesterol synthesis, has not been tested for safety during pregnancy and lactation.

New Molecular Medications

Mipomersen is an antisense oligonucleotide inhibitor of ApoB100. It binds to messenger RNA of ApoB100 resulting in its degradation and reduced of LDL and VLDL. Mipomersen, which has been used to treat HoFH, is classified as category B. It does not appear to cross the placenta and was undetectable in the fetal liver or kidney in mouse and rabbit studies. It is unknown whether mipomersen is excreted in breast milk; thus, women should be counseled about decision-making to discontinue the medication or stop breastfeeding.[72] This drug is no longer available in the United States.

Evolocumab

PCSK9 inhibitors are monoclonal antibodies that inhibit the binding of PCSK9 to the LDLR, thus increasing available LDLRs to process circulating LDL. Safety of these therapies has not been yet determined in pregnancy. However, a recent case report of evolocumab administered during 31 and 35 weeks gestation did not demonstrate any fetal complications.[73] Evolocumab crosses the placenta. Transfer of human antibody generally increases as pregnancy progresses with lowest exposure during organogenesis.[74] The presence of evolocumab in breast milk has not been studied.

OTHER ISSUES OF DYSLIPIDEMIA AND PREGNANCY

Several other conditions can lead to hyperlipidemia during pregnancy. Patients with autoimmune diseases can produce antibodies to apoproteins or any of the enzymes associated with lipid metabolism. GPIHBP1, the endothelial lipoprotein lipase anchoring protein, has a complicated 3 dimensional structure that makes it especially immunogenic. A patient with a lupuslike history was reported to have pregnancy-associated pancreatitis and a hypertriglyceridemic baby due to antibodies against GPIHBP1.[75] Clinicians should also be vigilant to exclude other common causes of dyslipidemia including hypothyroidism and the use of many medications.

CLINICS CARE POINTS

- Pregnancy increases triglyceride levels and may precipitate pancreatitis in patients with underlying genetic predisposition.
- Large systematic reviews of statin exposure during pregnancy have not consistently demonstrated fetal harm. Despite this, women exposed to statins during pregnancy should still undergo screening for possible congenital abnormalities.
- Generally, cholesterol-reducing medications should be avoided during pregnancy and lactation. When treatment is necessary for severe hypertriglyceridemia, resins and fish oil can be used.
- Lp(a) is a risk factor for coronary events and associated with some increased risk of pregnancy loss
- Data using newer liver genetic-based therapies and monoclonal antibody treatments in pregnancy are not yet available

DISCLOSURE

Dr I.J. Goldberg has received consulting fees from Arrowhead, Mammoth, and LG Pharmaceutical.

REFERENCES

1. Semenkovich CF, Goldberg IJ. Disorders of Lipid Metabolism. In: Melmed S, editor. Williams textbook of endocrinology. 14th edition. Philadelphia: Elsevier; 2020. p. 1581–621.
2. Bredefeld C, Peretti N, Hussain MM, et al. New Classification and Management of Abetalipoproteinemia and Related Disorders. Gastroenterology 2021;160(6): 1912–6.
3. Gagné C, Brun LD, Julien P, et al. Primary lipoprotein-lipase-activity deficiency: clinical investigation of a French Canadian population. Can Med Assoc J 1989; 140(4):405–11.
4. Belo L, Caslake M, Gaffney D, et al. Changes in LDL size and HDL concentration in normal and preeclamptic pregnancies. Atherosclerosis 2002;162(2):425–32.
5. Catov JM, Bodnar LM, Kip KE, et al. Early pregnancy lipid concentrations and spontaneous preterm birth. Am J Obstet Gynecol 2007;197(6):610.e1–7.
6. Palmisano BT, Zhu L, Stafford JM. Role of Estrogens in the Regulation of Liver Lipid Metabolism. Adv Exp Med Biol 2017;1043:227–56.
7. Zhu L, Brown WC, Cai Q, et al. Estrogen treatment after ovariectomy protects against fatty liver and may improve pathway-selective insulin resistance. Diabetes 2013;62(2):424–34.
8. Applebaum DM, Goldberg AP, Pykalisto OJ, et al. Effect of estrogen on postheparin lipolytic activity. Selective decline in hepatic triglyceride lipase. J Clin Invest 1977;59(4):601–8.
9. Hughes DL, Hughes A, White PB, et al. Acute pancreatitis in pregnancy: meta-analysis of maternal and fetal outcomes. Br J Surg 2021;109(1):12–4.
10. Kumar MP, Singh AK, Samanta J, et al. Acute pancreatitis in pregnancy and its impact on the maternal and foetal outcomes: A systematic review. Pancreatology 2022;22(2):210–8.
11. Berglund L, Brunzell JD, Goldberg AC, et al, Endocrine society. Evaluation and treatment of hypertriglyceridemia: an Endocrine Society clinical practice guideline. J Clin Endocrinol Metab 2012;97(9):2969–89.
12. Kim AS, Hakeem R, Abdullah A, et al. Therapeutic plasma exchange for the management of severe gestational hypertriglyceridaemic pancreatitis due to lipoprotein lipase mutation. Endocrinol Diabetes Metab Case Rep 2020;2020.
13. Safi F, Toumeh A, Abuissa Qadan MA, et al. Management of familial hypertriglyceridemia-induced pancreatitis during pregnancy with therapeutic plasma exchange: a case report and review of literature. Am J Ther 2014;21(5):e134–6.
14. Lee J, Goldberg IJ. Hypertriglyceridemia-induced pancreatitis created by oral estrogen and in vitro fertilization ovulation induction. J Clin Lipidol 2008; 2(1):63–6.
15. Reddy S, Ahmad Z. In vitro fertilization and hypertriglyceridemic pancreatitis: Case report. J Clin Lipidol 2022;16(4):417–22.
16. O'Byrne SM, Kako Y, Deckelbaum RJ, et al. Multiple pathways ensure retinoid delivery to milk: studies in genetically modified mice. Am J Physiol Endocrinol Metab 2010;298(4):E862–70.
17. Kleess LE, Janicic N. Severe Hypertriglyceridemia in Pregnancy: A Case Report and Review of the Literature. AACE Clin Case Rep 2019;5(2):e99–103.
18. Moulin P, Dufour R, Averna M, et al. Identification and diagnosis of patients with familial chylomicronaemia syndrome (FCS): Expert panel recommendations and proposal of an "FCS score". Atherosclerosis 2018;275:265–72.

19. Ginsberg HN, Goldberg IJ. Broadening the Scope of Dyslipidemia Therapy by Targeting APOC3 (Apolipoprotein C3) and ANGPTL3 (Angiopoietin-Like Protein 3). Arterioscler Thromb Vasc Biol 2023;43(3):388–98.
20. Motazacker MM, Pirruccello J, Huijgen R, et al. Advances in genetics show the need for extending screening strategies for autosomal dominant hypercholesterolaemia. Eur Heart J 2012;33(11):1360–6.
21. Blesa S, Vernia S, Garcia-Garcia A-B, et al. A New PCSK9 Gene Promoter Variant Affects Gene Expression and Causes Autosomal Dominant Hypercholesterolemia. J Clin Endocrinol Metabol 2008;93(9):3577–83.
22. Mousavi SA, Berge KE, Leren TP. The unique role of proprotein convertase subtilisin/kexin 9 in cholesterol homeostasis. J Intern Med 2009;266(6):507–19.
23. Cohen J, Pertsemlidis A, Kotowski IK, et al. Low LDL cholesterol in individuals of African descent resulting from frequent nonsense mutations in PCSK9. Nat Genet 2005;37(2):161–5.
24. Fasano T, Cefalu AB, Di Leo E, et al. A Novel Loss of Function Mutation of *PCSK9* Gene in White Subjects With Low-Plasma Low-Density Lipoprotein Cholesterol. Arterioscler Thromb Vasc Biol 2007;27(3):677–81.
25. Meng F-H, Liu S, Xiao J, et al. New Loss-of-Function Mutations in PCSK9 Reduce Plasma LDL Cholesterol. Arterioscler Thromb Vasc Biol 2023;43(7):1219–33.
26. Awan Z, Choi HY, Stitziel N, et al. APOE p.Leu167del mutation in familial hypercholesterolemia. Atherosclerosis 2013;231(2):218–22.
27. Cenarro A, Etxebarria A, de Castro-Orós I, et al. The p.Leu167del Mutation in APOE Gene Causes Autosomal Dominant Hypercholesterolemia by Downregulation of LDL Receptor Expression in Hepatocytes. J Clin Endocrinol Metabol 2016;101(5):2113–21.
28. Marduel M, Ouguerram K, Serre V, Bonnefont-Rousselot D, Marques-Pinheiro A, Erik Berge K, Devillers M, Luc G, Lecerf JM, Tosolini L, Erlich D, Peloso GM, Stitziel N, Nitchké P, Jaïs JP, French Research Network on ADH, Abifadel M, Kathiresan S, Leren TP, Rabès JP, Boileau C, Varret M. Description of a Large Family with Autosomal Dominant Hypercholesterolemia Associated with the *APOE* p.Leu167del Mutation. Hum Mutat 2013;34(1):83–7.
29. Khera AV, Won HH, Peloso GM, et al. Diagnostic Yield and Clinical Utility of Sequencing Familial Hypercholesterolemia Genes in Patients With Severe Hypercholesterolemia. J Am Coll Cardiol 2016;67(22):2578–89.
30. Hu P, Dharmayat KI, Stevens CAT, et al. Prevalence of Familial Hypercholesterolemia Among the General Population and Patients With Atherosclerotic Cardiovascular Disease. Circulation 2020;141(22):1742–59.
31. Nordestgaard BG, Chapman MJ, Humphries SE, et al, European Atherosclerosis Society Consensus Panel. Familial hypercholesterolaemia is underdiagnosed and undertreated in the general population: guidance for clinicians to prevent coronary heart disease: Consensus Statement of the European Atherosclerosis Society. Eur Heart J 2013;34(45):3478–90.
32. Beheshti SO, Madsen CM, Varbo A, et al. Worldwide Prevalence of Familial Hypercholesterolemia. J Am Coll Cardiol 2020;75(20):2553–66.
33. Orphanet Report Series. Prevalence and incidence of rare diseases: bibliographic data. Orphanet Report Series Rare diseases collection 2023.
34. Brown L, Ruel I, Baass A, et al. Homozygous Familial Hypercholesterolemia in Canada. JACC (J Am Coll Cardiol): Advances 2023;2(3):100309.
35. Mabuchi H, Nohara A, Noguchi T, et al, Hokuriku FH Study Group. Molecular genetic epidemiology of homozygous familial hypercholesterolemia in the Hokuriku district of Japan. Atherosclerosis 2011;214(2):404–7.

36. McGowan MP, Hosseini Dehkordi SH, Moriarty PM, et al. Diagnosis and Treatment of Heterozygous Familial Hypercholesterolemia. J Am Heart Assoc 2019;8(24).
37. An-Na C, Man-Li Y, Jeng-Hsiu H, et al. Alterations of serum lipid levels and their biological relevances during and after pregnancy. Life Sci 1995;56(26):2367–75.
38. Desoye G, Schweditsch MO, Pfeiffer KP, et al. Correlation of Hormones with Lipid and Lipoprotein Levels During Normal Pregnancy and Postpartum. J Clin Endocrinol Metabol 1987;64(4):704–12.
39. Herrera E, Lasunción MA, Gomez-Coronado D, et al. Role of lipoprotein lipase activity on lipoprotein metabolism and the fate of circulating triglycerides in pregnancy. Am J Obstet Gynecol 1988;158(6):1575–83.
40. Toleikyte I, Retterstøl K, Leren TP, et al. Pregnancy Outcomes in Familial Hypercholesterolemia. Circulation 2011;124(15):1606–14.
41. Pugh SJ, Schisterman EF, Browne RW, et al. Preconception maternal lipoprotein levels in relation to fecundability. Hum Reprod 2017;32(5):1055–63.
42. Schisterman EF, Mumford SL, Browne RW, et al. Lipid Concentrations and Couple Fecundity: The LIFE Study. J Clin Endocrinol Metabol 2014;99(8):2786–94.
43. Erqou S, Thompson A, Di Angelantonio E, et al. Apolipoprotein(a) Isoforms and the Risk of Vascular Disease. J Am Coll Cardiol 2010;55(19):2160–7.
44. Kamstrup PR, Tybjærg-Hansen A, Steffenson R, et al. Genetically Elevated Lipoprotein(a) and Increased Risk of Myocardial Infarction. JAMA 2009;301(22):2331.
45. Alonso R, Andres E, Mata N, et al, SAFEHEART Investigators. Lipoprotein(a) Levels in Familial Hypercholesterolemia. J Am Coll Cardiol 2014;63(19):1982–9.
46. Vuorio A, Watts GF, Schneider WJ, et al. Familial hypercholesterolemia and elevated lipoprotein(a): double heritable risk and new therapeutic opportunities. J Intern Med 2020;287(1):2–18.
47. Vuorio A, Watts GF, Kovanen PT. Lipoprotein(a) as a risk factor for calcific aortic valvulopathy in heterozygous familial hypercholesterolemia. Atherosclerosis 2019;281:25–30.
48. Boffa MB, Koschinsky ML. Lipoprotein (a): truly a direct prothrombotic factor in cardiovascular disease? JLR (J Lipid Res) 2016;57(5):745–57.
49. Boffa MB, Marar TT, Yeang C, et al. Potent reduction of plasma lipoprotein (a) with an antisense oligonucleotide in human subjects does not affect ex vivo fibrinolysis. JLR (J Lipid Res) 2019;60(12):2082–9.
50. Kamstrup PR, Tybjærg-Hansen A, Nordestgaard BG. Genetic Evidence That Lipoprotein(a) Associates With Atherosclerotic Stenosis Rather Than Venous Thrombosis. Arterioscler Thromb Vasc Biol 2012;32(7):1732–41.
51. Brighton TA, Eikelboom JW, Mann K, et al, ASPIRE Investigators. Low-Dose Aspirin for Preventing Recurrent Venous Thromboembolism. N Engl J Med 2012;367(21):1979–87.
52. Becattini C, Agnelli G, Schenone A, et al, WARFASA Investigators. Aspirin for Preventing the Recurrence of Venous Thromboembolism. N Engl J Med 2012;366(21):1959–67.
53. Matharu GS, Kunutsor SK, Judge A, et al. Clinical Effectiveness and Safety of Aspirin for Venous Thromboembolism Prophylaxis After Total Hip and Knee Replacement. JAMA Intern Med 2020;180(3):376.
54. Romagnuolo I, Sticchi E, Attanasio M, et al. Searching for a common mechanism for placenta-mediated pregnancy complications and cardiovascular disease: role of lipoprotein(a). Fertil Steril 2016;105(5):1287–12893 e3.

55. Tsimikas S, Karwatowska-Prokopczuk E, Gouni-Berthold I, et al, AKCEA-APOa-LRx Study Investigators. Lipoprotein(a) Reduction in Persons with Cardiovascular Disease. N Engl J Med 2020;382(3):244–55.

56. O'Donoghue ML, Rosenson RS, Gencer B, et al, OCEANa-DOSE Trial Investigators. Small Interfering RNA to Reduce Lipoprotein(a) in Cardiovascular Disease. N Engl J Med 2022;387(20):1855–64.

57. Luirink IK, Wiegman A, Kusters DM, et al. 20-Year Follow-up of Statins in Children with Familial Hypercholesterolemia. N Engl J Med 2019;381(16):1547–56.

58. Kastelein JJP, Ginsberg HN, Langslet G, et al. ODYSSEY FH I and FH II: 78 week results with alirocumab treatment in 735 patients with heterozygous familial hypercholesterolaemia. Eur Heart J 2015. ehv370-ehv.

59. Raal FJ, Rosenson RS, Reeskamp LF, et al, ELIPSE HoFH Investigators. Evinacumab for Homozygous Familial Hypercholesterolemia. N Engl J Med 2020;383(8):711–20.

60. Russi G. Severe dyslipidemia in pregnancy: The role of therapeutic apheresis. Transfus Apher Sci 2015;53(3):283–7.

61. Minsker DH, MacDonald JS, Robertson RT, et al. Mevalonate supplementation in pregnant rats suppresses the teratogenicity of mevinolinic acid, an inhibitor of 3-hydroxy-3-methylglutaryl-coenzyme a reductase. Teratology 1983;28(3):449–56.

62. Kusters DM, Lahsinoui HH, van de Post JAM, et al. Statin use during pregnancy: a systematic review and meta-analysis. Expet Rev Cardiovasc Ther 2012;10(3):363–78.

63. Zarek J, Koren G. The Fetal Safety of Statins: A Systematic Review and Meta-Analysis. J Obstet Gynaecol Can 2014;36(6):506–9.

64. Karalis DG, Hill AN, Clifton S, et al. The risks of statin use in pregnancy: A systematic review. Journal of Clinical Lipidology 2016;10(5):1081–90.

65. Newman CB, Preiss D, Tobert JA, et al, American Heart Association Clinical Lipidology, Lipoprotein, Metabolism and Thrombosis Committee, a Joint Committee of the Council on Atherosclerosis, Thrombosis and Vascular Biology and Council on Lifestyle and Cardiometabolic Health; Council on Cardiovascular Disease in the Young; Council on Clinical Cardiology; and Stroke Council. Statin Safety and Associated Adverse Events: A Scientific Statement From the American Heart Association. Arterioscler Thromb Vasc Biol 2019;39(2).

66. Hale TW, Krutsch K. Hale's Medications & Mothers' Milk 2023: A Manual of Lactational Pharmacology: Twentieth Edition2022.

67. Wong B, Ooi TC, Keely E. Severe gestational hypertriglyceridemia: A practical approach for clinicians. Obstet Med 2015;8(4):158–67.

68. Saadi HF, Kurlander DJ, Erkins JM, et al. Severe Hypertriglyceridemia and Acute Pancreatitis During Pregnancy: Treatment with Gemfibrozil. Endocr Pract 1999;5(1):33–6.

69. Jacobson TA, Maki KC, Orringer CE, et al, NLA Expert Panel. National Lipid Association Recommendations for Patient-Centered Management of Dyslipidemia: Part 2. Journal of clinical lipidology 2015;9(6 Suppl):S1–122.e1.

70. Dunstan JA, Simmer K, Dixon G, et al. Cognitive assessment of children at age 2½ years after maternal fish oil supplementation in pregnancy: a randomised controlled trial. Arch Dis Child Fetal Neonatal Ed 2008;93(1):F45–50.

71. Marquis JK, Dagher R, Baker BA, et al. Colesevelam hydrochloride does not cause maternal or fetal toxicity in rats and rabbits. Reprod Toxicol 2006;21(2):197–207.

72. McDonough A, Matura LA, Carroll D. New Pharmacologic Treatments for Familial Hypercholesterolemia. Nursing for Women's Health 2013;17(5):443–7.

73. Suzuki T, Tsurane K, Umemoto T, et al. PCSK9 inhibitor use during pregnancy in a case of familial hypercholesterolemia complicated with coronary artery disease. J Obstet Gynaecol Res 2024;50(1):128–32.
74. Palmeira P, Quinello C, Silveira-Lessa AL, et al. IgG Placental Transfer in Healthy and Pathological Pregnancies. Clin Dev Immunol 2012;2012:1–13.
75. Beigneux AP, Miyashita K, Ploug M, et al. Autoantibodies against GPIHBP1 as a Cause of Hypertriglyceridemia. N Engl J Med 2017;376(17):1647–58.

Moving?

Make sure your subscription moves with you!

To notify us of your new address, find your **Clinics Account Number** (located on your mailing label above your name), and contact customer service at:

Email: journalscustomerservice-usa@elsevier.com

800-654-2452 (subscribers in the U.S. & Canada)
314-447-8871 (subscribers outside of the U.S. & Canada)

Fax number: 314-447-8029

Elsevier Health Sciences Division
Subscription Customer Service
3251 Riverport Lane
Maryland Heights, MO 63043

*To ensure uninterrupted delivery of your subscription,
please notify us at least 4 weeks in advance of move.

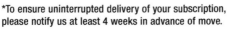

Printed and bound by CPI Group (UK) Ltd, Croydon, CR0 4YY

12/05/2025

01869427-0001